The Shoulder in Hemiplegia

The Shoulder in Hemiplegia

RENE CAILLIET, M.D.

Chairman and Professor
Department of Rehabilitation Medicine
University of Southern California
School of Medicine
Los Angeles, California

 F. A. DAVIS COMPANY, Philadelphia

Library of Congress Cataloging in Publication Data

Cailliet, Rene.
    The Shoulder in Hemiplegia

    Bibliography: p.
    Includes index.
        1. Shoulder--Paralysis.   2. Hemiplegics--Rehabilitation
3. Exercise therapy.   I. Title.   [DNLM:
1. Hemiplegia.   2. Shoulder.   WE810 C134h]
RC939.C35   617'.572   79-18598
ISBN 0-8036-1602-3

Preface

The hemiplegic patient can improve his ambulation, communication, balance, and self-care through treatment, but in the overall picture of functional return, the shoulder remains an enigma. It plays a vital role in self-care activities and is the basis of good hand function. It is vital in safe balance and ambulation and is often required for communication by the patient denied the return of speech. Good shoulder function is important for transfer activities or transport in a wheelchair. The shoulder may be the major site of severe and disabling pain and may be a contributing factor in ultimate loss of hand function.

In the early stage of adult hemiplegia, the shoulder is usually flaccid. It is solely supported by ligaments and capsule and may sublux. Irreparable damage to the surrounding tissues of the shoulder in this phase may decrease or even deny adequate function later.

Spasticity usually develops in the evolution of the completed stroke. In the spastic hemiplegic stroke, full range of motion is limited by spasticity, posture, righting reflexes, tonic neck reflexes, labyrinthine reflexes, group reflexes, sensory loss, and perceptual loss. Spasticity of the shoulder is not an isolated functional impairment. Secondary restrictions such as capsular thickening, ligamentous contracture, and tendon dysfunction become disabling factors. These soft tissue occurrences have been generally ignored or, at best, given inadequate consideration in the case of the hemiplegic shoulder.

The spastic posture of the shoulder in a standing or walking hemiplegic patient is usually that of adduction, internal rotation, and slight posterior protraction. The extended shoulder is accompanied by a flexed pattern of the remainder of the extremity with flexion of the elbow, wrist, and fingers, pronation of the forearm, and adduction of the thumb.

The hemiplegic shoulder position initially is the result of spastic muscular patterns with impairment of the agonist-antagonist neurologic balance. The hemiplegic shoulder pattern also is aggravated and maintained by secondary connective tissue contractures. These changes are noted very early in the evolution of the completed stroke. Spontaneous recovery has been documented by Twitchell and others but full recovery of the shoulder often lags far behind recovery of other aspects of the hemiplegic.

The hemiplegic patient may be markedly impaired but not afflicted with pain, except in the shoulder which may be severely painful, disabling, and recalcitrant to treatment. Treatment of the hemiplegic shoulder resides essentially in the domain of the physical therapist or occupational therapist or both and largely remains an enigma to them and the prescribing physician. In "Letters to the Editor" in the Journal of Physical Therapy a request was made for detailed clarification of "treating hemiplegic patients with range of motion exercises and arm positioning." This request was for definition of "range of motion exercises," clarification of exercise type as being passive or active, "Codman" type, or "P.N.F.," and verification of the significance of neurologic status in tone and sensation.[1,2]

Before any modality of treatment or technique of rehabilitation of the shoulder can be justified, basic functional anatomy must be clarified, abnormal neurophysiology explored, and concomitant pathologic changes ascertained. In this context the hemiplegic shoulder will be considered in this text.

The numerous theories of the neurophysiology of cerebrovascular disease and the techniques of rehabilitation cannot possibly be developed in detail. They will, however, be mentioned in their relation to the shoulder. The voluminous bibliography currently devoted to stroke will remain the reader's responsibility.

References

1. Dardier, E., and Reid, C.: Letters to the editor. Hemiplegia and painful shoulder. Phys. Ther. 52:1208, Nov. 1972.
2. Keelan, V.: Letters to the editor. Hemiplegia and painful shoulder. Phys. Ther. 52:1209, Nov. 1972.

Contents

1. **Hemiplegia**   1

   Neuropathy   2

   Upper Extremity Function   4

   Summary   8

   References   9

2. **Functional Anatomy of the Shoulder**   11

   Glenohumeral Joint   11

   Suprahumeral Joint   18

   Suspensory Ligaments   20

   Coracohumeral Ligament   20

   Musculature of the Glenohumeral Joint   20

   Bursae   26

   Nerve Supply to Shoulder   27

   Glenohumeral Movement   30

   Scapular Movement   36

   Scapulohumeral Movement   42

   Acromioclavicular and Sternoclavicular
        Joints   44

   Composite Shoulder Girdle Movements   47

   Biceps Mechanism   49

   Summary   53

   References   53

3. **Flaccid Stage**   55
    Flail Extremity   55
    Subluxation of the Shoulder   63
    Summary   68
    References   70

4. **Spastic Stage**   73
    Techniques of Muscle Reeducation   79
    References   86

5. **The Painful Shoulder**   89
    Radiologic Examination   92
    Acromioclavicular Lesion   95
    Bicipital Tendinitis   95
    Coracoiditis   96
    Brachial Plexus Traction   98
    Diagnosis   99
    Treatment   99
    Summary   106
    References   106

6. **Shoulder-Hand-Finger Syndrome**   107
    Theories of Etiology of Pain   115
    Treatment   115
    References   119

7. **Brachial Plexus Injury**   121

    Bibliography   123

    Index   127

List of Illustrations

1. Central nervous system   3
2. Estimate of spontaneous recovery from stroke   5
3. Stages of recovery from stroke   6
4. Flexor synergy of upper extremity   8
5. Composite drawing of the should girdle   12
6. Acromiocoracoid arch   13
7. Scapula   14
8. Congruous-incongruous joints   15
9. Glenohumeral synovial capsule   16
10. Capsular action during glenohumeral movement   17
11. Anterior capsule and the glenohumeral ligaments   19
12. Coracohumeral ligament   21
13. Rotator cuff   21
14. Sites of muscular origin and insertion upon the scapula and the humerus   22
15. Supraspinatus muscle and the infraspinatus muscle   23
16. Function of supraspinatus muscle   24
17. Subscapularis muscle   25
18. Subacromial bursa   27
19. Nerve supply of the shoulder   28
20. Circulation of the tendons of the cuff: the critical zone   29
21. Blood circulation   29
22. Capsular-passive cuff support   30
23. Planes of arm movement   31
24. Deltoid muscle and its isolated function   32

25. Abduction angle of deltoid   33
26. Glenohumeral movement of arm abduction   35
27. Combined cuff and deltoid action upon
        the glenohumeral articulation   36
28. Influence of humeral rotation upon abduction
        range of the glenohumeral joint   37
29. Scapular musculature: rotators   38
30. Downward rotators of the scapula   40
31. Pectoralis major   41
32. Scapulohumeral rhythm (Codman)   43
33. Deltoid action upon the glenohumeral joint   44
34. Action of the coracoclavicular ligaments
        upon the acromioclavicular joint   45
35. Scapular elevation resulting from clavicular
        rotation   46
36. Sternoclavicular joint   47
37. Muscles acting upon the clavicle   48
38. Accessory movement of the scapulohumeral
        rhythm other than the glenohumeral movement 50
39. Biceps mechanism   52
40. Extension and flexion pattern of the upper
        extremity in neck extension and flexion   57
41. Entire upper extremity enclosed within
        an air-inflated splint   59
42. Patient supine, extremity is gradually
        raised to overhead position   60
43. Passive exercise, patient tries to hold
        extremity in various positions   61
44. Mobilization of the shoulder to regain joint play   62
45. In sitting position, supporting weight
        on affected side   64
46. Mechanism of glenohumeral subluxation   66
47. Scapular depression   66
48. Spastic medial scapular muscles   67
49. Shoulder slings   68
50. Rood sling   69
51. Proposed design for prevention of subluxation   69
52. Wheel chair arm sling   70
53. Denial demonstrated by patient   77
54. Patient crawling with weight-bearing
        on affected arm   81
55. Patient sitting and leaning on affected arm   82

56. Rhythmic stabilization technique to increase
shoulder joint range of motion 83
57. Alternating cycle of rhythmic stabilization 84
58. Five Ds resulting from pain 90
59. Circulation to the critical zone of the
supraspinatus tendon 91
60. Sites of tissue pain 92
61. Roentgenographic changes in shoulder
dysfunction: cysts in the tuberosities
of the humerus 93
62. Stages of degeneration 95
63. Adhesive capsulitis 98
64. Injection technique for intraarticular
arthrogram and brisement treatment 101
65. Techniques for injection treatment of
supraspinatus tendinitis 101
66. Suprascapular nerve block 102
67. Postoperative bracing 103
68. Home exercises for painful restricted shoulder 104
69. Shoulder exercises 105
70. Venous lymphatic pumps of the upper extremity 108
71. Normal flexion-extension of
metacarpophalangeal joints 109
72. Finger changes in hand-shoulder syndrome 110
73. Hand patterns 111
74. Sequences leading to frozen shoulder-
hand-finger syndrome 112
75. Technique of stellate ganglion or brachial
plexus block 117
76. Removal of finger edema 118
77. Antigravity treatment of edematous extremity 119

CHAPTER 1

Hemiplegia

Stroke syndrome is caused by vascular lesions of the brain, such as hemorrhage, thrombosis, embolism, or spasm. The resultant neurologic impairment depends on the specific site of vascular occulsion of the brain, size of brain insult, and laterality. Impairment may be singular, multiple, or diffuse and involve sensory or motor loss. Frequently the neurologic impairment is unilateral and marked by hemiplegia or hemiparesis. The physician caring for the patient with the completed stroke should concentrate on rehabilitation and direct his attention to recovery or improvement of function and prevention of any factor that adds to greater disability. Present evidence has shown that drugs and surgical intervention have not as yet proven to be of great functional value. Obviously, concomitant with rehabilitation efforts all factors that lead to further disease and pathology need to be minimized. Among these factors are concurrent heart disease, hypertension, polycythemia, diabetes mellitus, and numerous conditions leading to central nervous system hypoxia.

In his dissertation on rehabilitation of the adult hemiplegic, Peszczynski discussed "special techniques" of rehabilitation. He stated, "It would be wise to consider most of them as working hypotheses for further research and observation."[1] He questioned the separation of concentrated motor performance learning from

1

automatic recovery or from substitution for improved motor function. He also challenged the efficacy of gradually and ultimately developing voluntary activity through mass reflex movement or superimposed sensory stimulation. The advisability of concentrating on single motions as opposed to more complex movement also has not been universally clarified and confirmed.

Some reeducation of motor function has been evidenced in most patients undergoing rehabilitation treatment. Improvement in function has been far greater and faster in patients receiving treatment than in patients allowed to merely undergo spontaneous recovery. Furthermore, it is possible that a great portion of functional recovery is enhanced by preventing secondary complications such as contracture, pain, joint limitation, and decrease of motivation. Many latent neuropsychologic pathways probably become activated by special techniques of therapy using sensory stimulation, basic reflexes, and repeated efforts, but these remain to be documented, verified, and standardized for general use.

There is a wide spectrum of opinion regarding the basis as well as the value of many of the current rehabilitation efforts. Birch and associates felt that rehabilitation of the hemiplegic patient is a problem of training him to utilize his residual motor abilities.[2] At the other end of the spectrum, Kabat claims "new pathways" can be developed in the extrapyramidal tracts by special treatment techniques.[3] Kottke poses the usual question "Are techniques of facilitation and inhibition of value to increased neuromuscular function following stroke?"[4]

At present none of these questions can be specifically and objectively answered, but neurophysiologic concepts merit further study and newer techniques of therapy must be developed, tested, and clarified.

NEUROPATHOLOGY

In the evolution of the central nervous system, as higher centers of complex patterns develop, the grosser patterns of the lower centers are inhibited. In damage to the central nervous

2

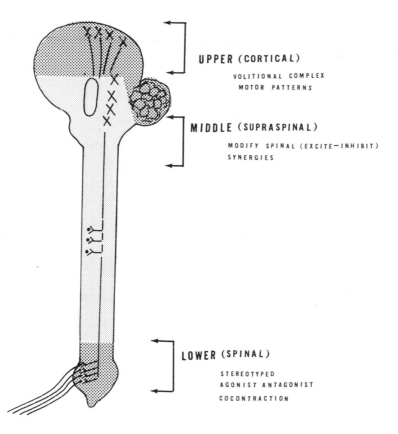

UPPER (CORTICAL)

VOLITIONAL COMPLEX
MOTOR PATTERNS

MIDDLE (SUPRASPINAL)

MODIFY SPINAL (EXCITE—INHIBIT)
SYNERGIES

LOWER (SPINAL)

STEREOTYPED
AGONIST ANTAGONIST
COCONTRACTION

FIGURE 1. Central nervous system.

system, as in stroke, the higher centers containing the complex patterns and the facility for the inhibition of massive gross patterns lose control and the uncontrolled, or partially controlled, stereotyped patterns of the middle and lower centers emerge. In essence, there are no pathologic reflexes but merely normal stereotyped lower spinal and middle supraspinal reflexes that are no longer activated, modified, or inhibited. Jackson[5] postulated that the higher centers or cortical regulators modify the lower centers by gradually developing complex patterns of motor activity.

In normal people, sensory activation of internuncial motor neurons must be present to enable the central nervous system to

3

react to cerebral volitional activities. Also, the internuncial pool of the subcortical center must be inhibited to prevent involuntary activities. In the hemiplegic interaction and control are interrupted and most reeducation techniques are aimed at regaining these two functions.

UPPER EXTREMITY FUNCTION

The upper extremity, and in particular the shoulder, exemplifies these concepts. Specific motor function volitionally originating in the upper cortical centers, such as fine precise finger movements, is made possible by precise positioning of the shoulder. In hemiplegia the upper centers are lost and thus fine precise movement of the hand and shoulder are partially or completely lost. In severe central nervous system damage, spasticity results and reflex synergies emerge.

There are numerous factors that influence upper extremity function after a stroke:

1. Natural sequential return of function
2. Spasticity
3. Primitive reflex pattern synergies
4. Apraxia
5. Contracture
6. Peripheral sensory deficit
7. Perceptual involvement
8. Intellectual impairment

The upper extremity is more severely involved in all types of strokes, except when the anterior cerebral artery is involved. Upper extremity recovery is usually not as complete as is the functional recovery of the lower extremity. The sequence of recovery was documented by Twitchell in 1951.[6]

0 hours
1. Immediately after hemiplegia there is a total loss of voluntary function with loss or decrease of tendon reflexes.

2. Flaccidity or decrease in resistance to passive movement occurs.

48 hours 3. Deep tendon reflexes increase on the involved side with possible clonus. In the upper extremity this increase is first noted in the finger flexors and the forearm with marked resistance of the adductors and flexors of the upper arm.

3–31 days 4. Clasp knife phenomenon appears in elbow flexors.

Return of voluntary function, as stated by Twitchell, usually begins with flexion of the shoulder in the first 6 to 33 days, followed by development of total flexor synergy spreading distally in the extremity. These synergistic patterns are markedly influ-

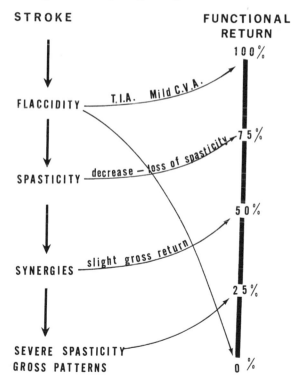

FIGURE 2.   Estimate of spontaneous recovery from stroke.

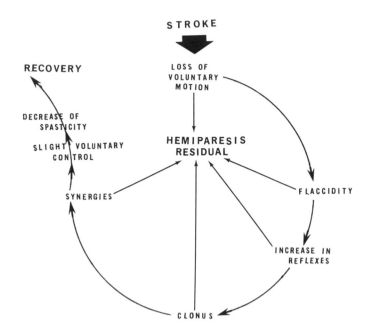

FIGURE 3. Stages of recovery from stroke.

enced by proprioceptive stimuli. Gradual voluntary control return is accompanied by disappearance of flexor synergy and a decrease in spasticity. Complete motor return may occur with only residual increased deep tendon reflexes and easy fatigability or with varying degrees of residual paresis, weakness, spotty spasticity, or residual flexor synergies.

Brunnstrom[7] designated the following stages observed in recovery which could be the basis of prognosis or evaluation.

Stage I   Flaccidity.

Stage II   Gradual development of spasticity with beginning of synergies.

Stage III Increase in spasticity with some voluntary control of synergies if patient is improving.

Stage IV   Decline of spasticity with increasing control of components of the synergies. Recovery may end at this stage with persistence of synergies or with partial decrease of total synergies.

Stage V Synergies no longer control motor acts.

Stage VI Development of individual joint movement with early coordination.

In the patients who undergo spontaneous motor recovery,[8] 40 percent regain full motion of the arm. In these, there is initial return within the first two weeks with the shoulder, elbow, and hand all showing signs of recovery during the same week. In those who ultimately progress to a full return of function, recovery will usually be completed within four weeks and always within three months. Forty percent regain partial movement with continuing improvement up to the seventh month. Twenty percent show no return of function.

Full return of motion is noted mostly in the elbow, less in the hand, and *least in the shoulder*. Even in full recovery of the upper extremity, shoulder impairment can often be noticed with residual limited full overhead extension of the arm. Full range of motion of the arm and hand does not assure full functional return as there may be associated apraxia, dystonia, sensory loss, loss of coordination, perceptual loss, and intellectual impairment.

Carroll[9] found that only 4 percent of hemiplegic patients regained complete neurologic recovery of the upper extremity. Carroll claimed that "no return of function within a week" usually meant there would not be a return to full *use* of the extremity. "Use" here implies serviceable function including sensation and coordination but this author merely was concerned with hand-finger activities and did not consider shoulder function. Sensory function may often return in a matter of time.[10] Prognosis is more guarded if disturbance of two point discrimination persists. This impairment indicates parietal cortical damage with probable perceptive loss.

In the sequence of evolution of neurologic sequelae of hemipareses, the upper extremity develops consistent synergistic patterns: flexion of upper extremities, flexion at elbow, adduction of shoulder, internal rotation of shoulder, wrist and fingers flexed, forearm pronated. The development of these synergies results

7

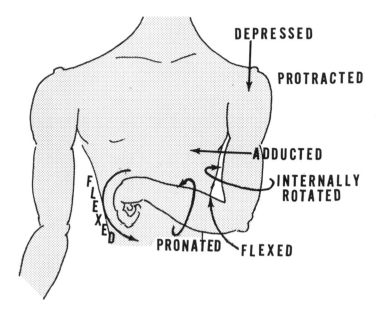

FIGURE 4.   Flexor synergy of upper extremity.

when the higher centers are ablated thus removing the pyramidal and extrapyramidal control. The labyrinth becomes the controller of posture through the basal ganglia and tonic neck reflexes. Any motion of the head in relationship to the horizontal plane will modify the basic labyrinthine posture. The basal ganglia are stimulated via the effect of gravity on the otoliths of the saccule and utricle of the inner ear.

The supraspinal tonic neck reflexes become activated by rotation of the head. Rotation of the head causes extension of the upper extremity on the side toward which the head is rotated and flexion of the extremity in the opposite extremity. Extension causes extensor tonus of the upper extremity whereas flexion (of the neck) enhances the flexor pattern of the upper extremity.[11]

SUMMARY

The natural evolution of the stroke has predictable stages of progression and improvement. Many variables are interposed

8

that modify these stages, influence their occurrence, and influence the ultimate extent of recovery or residual impairment. Not all these variables are amenable to therapeutic approaches.

Shoulder impairment does not conform to all the stages of progression nor to the stages of recovery from stroke. Its participation in the various stages of progression is not uniform and its presence in the stages of recovery is variable. Its degree of recovery and its response to therapy is also unpredictable.

There are complications in the recovery of shoulder function that justify its being studied separately. Subluxation is unique in the stroke involvement of the shoulder. Pain in the shoulder is more prevalent than in other aspects of the extremities. Contracture with limitation of motion is prevalent. Its participation in the patterns of spasticity and synergy is not always uniform nor predictable.

Because of its function as an incongruous joint with so many articulations and muscles involved, it is a complex joint to evaluate and treat. The normal neuromuscular patterns are complicated hence they are doubly so in the hemiplegic state.

The shoulder is involved in all aspects of the natural progression of the stroke: the flaccid stage, spastic stage, development of the synergies, and the stages of recovery. Complications include subluxation, contracture, pain, and dystrophic changes. The hemiplegic shoulder, admittedly an enigma to the therapist, remains only partially understood but many facets of its impairment are being pieced together into a meaningful pattern.

REFERENCES

1. Peszczynski, M.: The status of research on recovery of function in hemiplegia. Presented at Fifteenth Scientific Session of the French Society of Prevention and Social Medicine, Paris, Sept. 1967.
2. Birch, H. D., Proctor, F., Bortner, M., et al.: Perception in hemiplegia. Judgment of vertical and horizontal by hemiplegic patient. Arch. Phys. Med. 41:19, 1960.
3. Kabat, H.: Studies on neuromuscular dysfunction XI. New principles of neuromuscular reeducation. Permante Found. Med. Bull. 5:111, 1947.
4. Kottke, F.: Neurophysiologic therapy for stroke, in Licht, S. (ed.): Stroke and Its Rehabilitation. Elizabeth Licht Publisher, New Haven, 1975.

5. Jackson, J. H.: On some implications of dissolution of the nervous system. Med. Press Circular 2:411, 1882.
6. Twitchell, T. E.: The restoration of motor function following hemiplegia. Brain 74:443, 1951.
7. Brunnstrom, S.: Movement Therapy in Hemiplegia: A Neurophysiological Approach. Harper and Row, New York, 1970.
8. Bard, G., and Hirschberg, G.: Recovery of voluntary motion in upper extremity following hemiplegia. Arch. Phys. Med. Rehabil. 45:567, 1965.
9. Carroll, D.: Hand function in hemiplegia. J. Chronic Dis. 18:493, 1965.
10. Van Buskirk, C., and Webster, D.: Prognostic value of sensory deficit in rehabilitation of hemiplegia. Neurology 5:407, 1955.
11. Fielding, J. W., Burstein, A. H., Frankel, V. H.: The nuchal ligament. Spine 1:3, March 1976.

CHAPTER 2

Functional Anatomy
of the Shoulder

The shoulder is essentially a composite of seven joints, all moving synchronously and incumbent upon each other to insure complete pain-free movement. The term "shoulder girdle" is a preferable term and implies "thoracoscapulohumeral articulation." All seven joints of the shoulder girdle have significance in ultimately placing the hand in a proper functional position.

The humeroscapular portion of the girdle attaches to the vertebral column via the acromioclavicular joint, then, proximally, via the sternoclavicular joint, the costosternal joint, and ultimately the costovertebral joints. These four joints have a unique function and permit motion as well as maintaining the arm at the person's side. They will be given consideration in subsequent pages.

GLENOHUMERAL JOINT

The glenohumeral joint is the major site of movement of the shoulder girdle. This is joint 1 in Figure 5. The articulation comprises the glenoid fossa of the scapula and the head of the humerus. Overhanging the glenohumeral joint but indirectly related to its function is the suprahumeral joint which is essentially a functional joint rather than a true articulation. This "joint" is

11

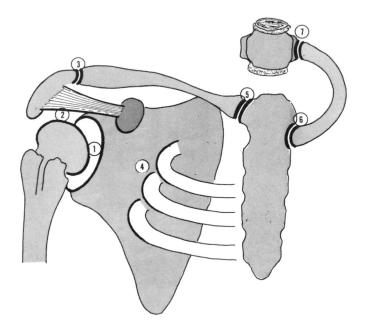

FIGURE 5. Composite drawing of the shoulder girdle.
1 = Glenohumeral   5 = Sternoclavicular
2 = Suprahumeral   6 = Costosternal
3 = Acromioclavicular   7 = Costovertebral
4 = Scapulocostal

formed by the overhanging acromion and the coracoacromial ligament (Fig. 6). The glenohumeral joint may also be termed the scapulohumeral joint in that it is the "true" joint between the humerus and the scapula.

The scapula or "shoulder blade" (Fig. 7) lies on the posterior surface of the thoracic cage, with its ventral surface concave corresponding to the convex surface of the rib cage. The only attachments to the thorax and spinal column other than via the acromioclavicular joint are muscular. The dorsal surface of the scapula is divided by the spine, a horizontal bony ridge that extends laterally past the glenoid fossa ending in a bulbous end, the acromial process. This process overhangs the head of the humerus, is the site of attachment to the clavicle (the acromioclavicular joint), and receives the fibers of the coracoacromial

12

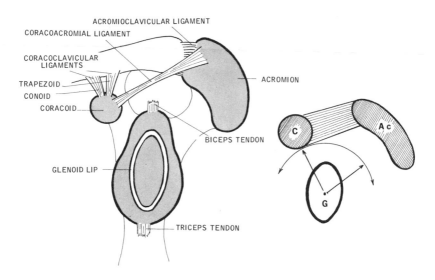

FIGURE 6. The acromiocoracoid arch. The diagram depicts the shape of the glenoid fossa and its relationship to the acromial process, the coracoid process, and the coracoacromial ligament. In essence this diagram shows the socket of the *glenohumeral* joint and also portrays the relationship of the *suprahumeral* joint.

ligament. The acromion and the coracoacromial ligament form part of the arch overlying the suprahumeral joint (Fig. 6).

The glenoid fossa, the socket of the glenohumeral joint, is located on the anterosuperior angle of the scapula, midway between and below the acromion and the coracoid process. The glenoid fossa is shallow and ovoid and faces anteriorly, laterally, and upward (Figs. 6 and 7). The direction upward has clinical significance in furnishing stability to the glenohumeral joint.

Surrounding the perimeter of the fossa and deepening the cup is a fibrous lip known as the glenoid labrum. This lip, originally considered to be fibrocartilage,[1] contains no cartilage but is primarily fibrous tissue, a redundant fold of the anterior capsule.[2] This fold, and apparently the labrum, disappears as the humerus is externally rotated.

There is a marked discrepancy between the surface area and the curvature of the glenoid fossa and the convex surface of the humeral head. The angular sphere of the humeral head is 180°

13

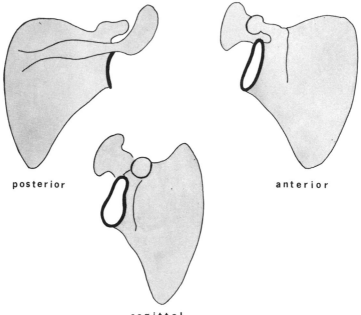

posterior   anterior

sagittal

FIGURE 7. The scapula. The posterior, anterior, and sagittal views of the scapula are shown. The spine of the scapula seen on the posterior view divides the blade into the supra- and infraspinatus fossae, from which originate the muscles that also bear these names. The sagittal view is more graphically seen in Figure 2, which depicts the relationship of the glenoid fossa to the overhanging acromial process and the medially located coracoid process. Note the angle of the glenoid fossa, facing laterally, anteriorly, and *upwards*.

and that of the glenoid cavity 60°. Two thirds of the humeral head is not covered by the glenoid.

The glenohumeral joint is an incongruous joint and thus sacrifices stability for mobility. The humeral head, in this incongruous relationship, moves by gliding about a moving axis rather than by rotation about a fixed axis (Fig. 8). The muscles that mobilize the humeral head must also afford stability. The capsule must be more redundant than is needed on a congruous or ball and socket joint. From a purely skeletal aspect, abduction to 120° should be possible in the glenohumeral joint, also greater internal and external rotation, but this movement is restricted by soft tissue:

14

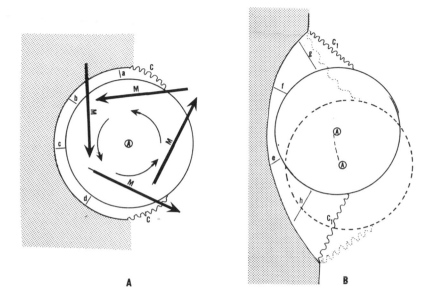

FIGURE 8.   Congruous-incongruous joints. *A*, In a *congruous* joint the concave, convex surfaces are symmetrical. The articular surfaces are equidistant from each other at all points along their circumference (a = b = c = d, etc.). In rotation, movement occurs about a fixed axis Ⓐ. Muscular action M is that of symmetrical movement about this fixed axis and is needed for motion, not stability. The depth of the concave surface gives the joint stability. The capsule (C) has symmetrical elongation. *B*, *Incongruous* joints have asymmetrical articulatory surfaces. The concave surface is elongated and the convex more circular, thus the distance between them varies at each point (g > f > e < h). As the joint moves, the axis of rotation Ⓐ shifts and joint movement is that of gliding rather than rolling. Therefore, muscles must slide the joint and simultaneously maintain stability. The capsule C, varies in its elongation at all levels of movement. The glenohumeral joint is an incongruous joint.

ligament capsule and muscles. Restraint of joint motion can occur in all directions or in one plane: in the glenohumeral joint it varies in numerous planes. Restraint may be structural (physiologic) or protective (pathologic) from spasm or inflammatory tissue changes.

When shoulder muscles are removed leaving the humerus attached to the scapula only by the capsule and ligaments, the head of the humerus can be drawn one-third inch away from its socket. In the adducted position, the capsule becomes tight and prevents downward displacement of the humerus.

15

Glenohumeral Capsule

The capsule of the glenohumeral joint is an extremely thin-walled, spacious container that attaches around the entire perimeter of the glenoid rim. The capsule arises from the glenoid fossa and inserts around the anatomic neck of the humerus (Fig. 9). There is a synovial lining throughout that blends with the hyaline cartilage of the head of the humerus but fails to reach the cartilage of the glenoid fossa (Fig. 9B). The fibrous capsule attaches from just proximal to the margin of the glenoid fossa to the anatomic neck of the humerus.

The long head of the biceps tendon attaches to the superior aspect of the glenoid fossa (see Fig. 6). It invaginates the capsule but does not enter the synovial cavity. The biceps tendon is thus

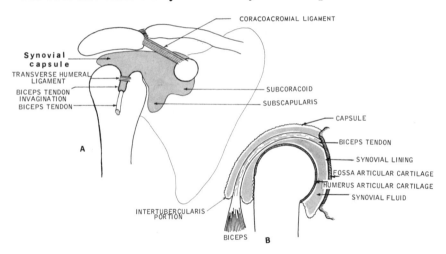

FIGURE 9. Glenohumeral synovial capsule. *A*, The spacious capsule covering the entire humeral head. The invagination of the capsule accompanying the biceps tendon down the bicipital groove passes under the transverse humeral ligament at the level of the point of attachment of the pectoralis major muscle to the shaft of the humerus. The subscapularis and subcoracoid pouches of the capsule contain synovial fluid and are in direct continuity with the major capsule. These pouches are clearly seen in dye arthrograms. *B*, The *intra*capsular *extra*synovial invagination of the long head of the biceps tendon as it proceeds to attach to the superior rim of the glenoid fossa. The synovial lining attaches to the articular cartilage of the head of the humerus but attaches to the glenoid fossa at a distance from the rim of the glenoid cartilage.

16

intracapsular but remains extrasynovial. The capsule folds and incorporates the biceps tendon down into the intertubercular sulcus of the humerus and ends blindly at a site on the humerus opposite the insertion of the pectoralis major muscle (Fig. 9A).[3]

With the arm hanging loosely in a dependent position at the side, the upper portion of the capsule is taut, and the inferior portion, the axillary fold, is loose and pleated (Fig. 10). The opposite situation exists when the arm is fully abducted. Here

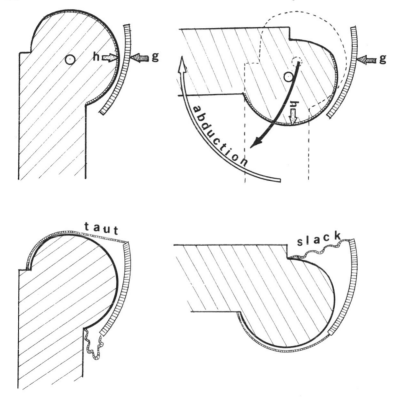

FIGURE 10. Capsular action during glenohumeral movement. The upper figure depicts the "gliding" joint motion between the head of the humerus and the glenoid fossa. The arcs of both joint surfaces differ and thus form an incongruous joint surface relationship. The lower left figure shows the arm dependent with the superior portion of the capsule taut, which prevents downward movement. The lower right figure shows the arm abducted, which relaxes the superior portion of the capsule and causes the inferior portion to become taut. In the half-abducted arm both superior and inferior capsules are slack, which position is thus one of instability of the glenohumeral joint.

the inferior portion becomes taut and the superior portion pleated. The tautness of the superior capsule with the arm dependent prevents downward dislocation of the arm, and the laxity of the capsule permits the gliding motion of the glenohumeral joint.

Rotation of the arm around its longitudinal axis (turning the arm in and out and to and from the trunk while dependent) has the same effect of tautness and laxity upon the capsule, anteriorly and posteriorly. The anterior portion of the capsule is reinforced by the superior, middle, and inferior glenohumeral ligaments. These ligaments are actually pleated horizontal folds of the anterior capsule in a fan-shaped appearance in front of the glenohumeral joint. Glenohumeral ligaments (superior, middle, and inferior) pass obliquely from the front and lower part of the anatomic neck of the humerus and go medially and upward to attach (converge) on the supraglenoid tubercle. The inferior band contributes to the anterior portion of the glenoid fossa. The superior band parallels the biceps tendon attached to the humerus and converges toward the glenoid rim, some distance in from the edge of the fossa, to attach on the anterosuperior portion of the glenoid and the adjacent bone (Fig. 11). These ligaments restrict external rotation of the humerus.

There is a recess or pouch in the anterior capsule due to the looseness of the capsule. The capsule is actually loose enough to permit the humerus to be drawn as much as 3 cm. from the fossa. An opening usually exists between the superior and middle glenohumeral ligaments (folds) termed the foramen of Weitbrecht, which is merely covered by a thin layer of capsule, or may be open as a communication between the joint capsule and the subscapular recess. The anterior pouch, due to capsular laxity and the foramen of Weitbrecht, assumes significance in dislocations of the humerus.[4]

THE SUPRAHUMERAL JOINT

The suprahumeral joint is not a joint in the true definition: an articulation, more or less movable, between two or more bones.[5]

18

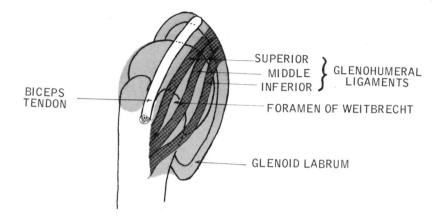

BICEPS
TENDON

SUPERIOR
MIDDLE
INFERIOR
} GLENOHUMERAL
LIGAMENTS

FORAMEN OF WEITBRECHT

GLENOID LABRUM

FIGURE 11. Anterior capsule and the glenohumeral ligaments. The glenohumeral *ligaments* that reinforce the anterior joint capsule are mere folds of the capsule. Three in number, they are fan-shaped, attach from the humerus, and converge towards the glenoid rim. The foramen of Weitbrecht may be covered by a thin layer or may be open as a communication between the joint space and the subscapular recess.

The suprahumeral joint is more a protective articulation between the head of the humerus and an arch formed by a broad, triangular ligament connecting the acromial process and the coracoid process (see Fig. 6).

The coracoacromial arch prevents trauma from above to the glenohumeral joint or to the head of the humerus and also prevents upward dislocation of the humerus. Its proximity to the humerus in its inner aspect mechanically limits abduction of the humerus in the coronal plane.

The suprahumeral articulation is bounded within by the glenoid cavity, superiorly and slightly posteriorly by the acromial process, anteriorly and medially by the coracoid process, and above by the coracoacromial ligament. The humeral head lies under this hood.

Within the suprahumeral joint are found portions of the subacromial bursa, the subcoracoid bursa, the supraspinatus muscle and its tendon, the superior portion of the glenohumeral capsule, a portion of the biceps tendon, and the interposed loose connective tissue. Many sensitive tissues are enclosed within this small area.[6,7]

19

SUSPENSORY LIGAMENTS

The suspensory ligaments, so termed by DiPalma[1] are the coracohumeral ligament and the cuff muscles. These ligaments prevent the arm from falling downward, but DiPalma claims that severance of the ligament does not affect glenohumeral movement.

CORACOHUMERAL LIGAMENT

This ligament passes from the coracoid process down to the humerus parallel to the biceps tendon between the supraspinatus muscle and the subscapularis. It retracts (shortens) with inward rotation of the arm and plays a part in the internally rotated "frozen shoulder" and probably is involved in most limited painful shoulders. The coracohumeral ligament attaches to the anatomic neck of the humerus beside the lesser and greater tubercle, Its posterior fibers blend with the capsule. This ligament resists lateral rotation and abduction (Fig. 12). Downward dislocation of the shoulder is prevented by (1) slope of the glenoid fossa, (2) tightening of the superior position of the capsule and the coracohumeral ligament, (3) the supraspinatus muscle of the cuff.

MUSCULATURE OF THE GLENOHUMERAL JOINT

The strength of the shoulder joint depends upon muscles and their tendons, not upon the bony configuration nor ligaments. These tendons are accessory dynamic ligaments. The supraspinatus fuses intimately with the underlying fibrous capsule. The infraspinatus and subscapularis muscles and their tendons fuse less intimately. In abduction the triceps and the teres major contract the interior capsule.

Four of the nine muscles related to the glenohumeral joint are prime movers that collectively form the *musculotendinous cuff* or more commonly the *rotator cuff* (Fig. 13). The muscles com-

20

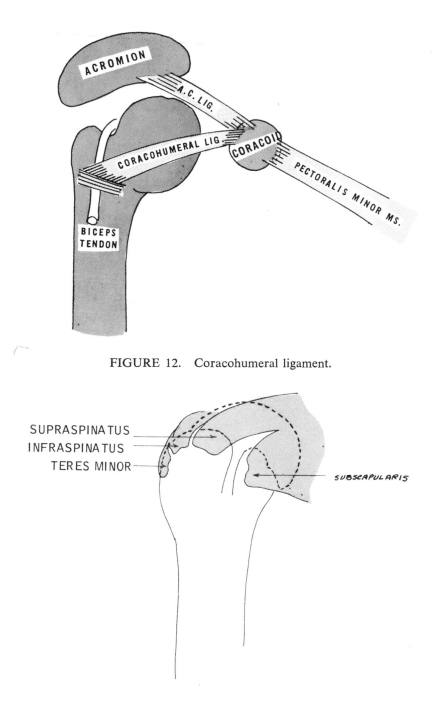

FIGURE 12.   Coracohumeral ligament.

SUPRASPINATUS
INFRASPINATUS
TERES MINOR

SUBSCAPULARIS

FIGURE 13.   Rotator cuff.

prising the rotator cuff are the supraspinatus, infraspinatus, teres minor, and the subscapularis muscles. Through the attachment of their conjoined tendon upon the humerus, they abduct and rotate the arm internally or externally. The cuff muscles act as rotators in two planes: (1) movement of abduction and adduction in the coronal plane and (2) rotation about the longitudinal axis of the humerus in internal and external rotation of the arm. Both are inextricably related in scapulohumeral movement. (Fig. 14).

The supraspinatus muscle originates from the supraspinatus fossa of the scapula above the spine of the scapula (Fig. 15) on its posterior surface. It passes laterally under the coracoacromial ligament and attaches to the greater tuberosity of the humeral head (Fig. 16). As the supraspinatus progresses to its point of

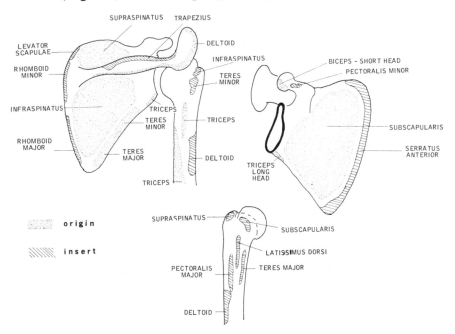

FIGURE 14. Sites of muscular origin and insertion upon the scapula and the humerus. All the muscles that perform shoulder girdle function are shown here. The dotted areas indicate the area from which the muscles originate, and the thatched areas represent areas to which the muscles or their tendons insert.

22

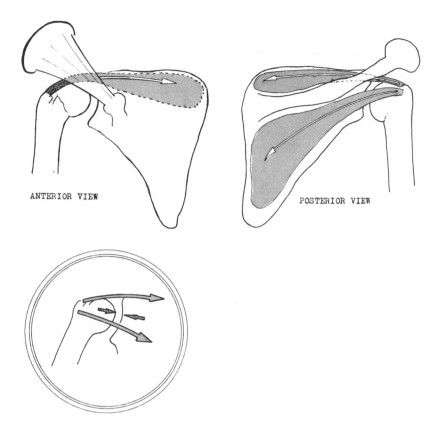

FIGURE 15. Supraspinatus muscle and the infraspinatus muscle.
Anterior view, The supraspinatus muscle originates from the supraspinatus fossa of the scapula and passes laterally under the coracohumeral
ligament to attach upon the greater tuberosity of the humerus. *Posterior
view,* The infraspinatus muscle originates from the infraspinatus fossa
and inserts upon the greater tuberosity just below the insertion of the
supraspinatus tendon. The combined action of these two muscles (shown
in insert) brings the head of the humerus against the glenoid fossa in a
slightly "downward" direction.

attachment, it passes superiorly to the axis of rotation of the abducting arm and anterior to the axis of rotation of the inwardly/
outwardly rotating arm. Thus, it (1) seats the head of the humerus into the glenoid fossa, (2) slightly abducts the humerus, and
(3) externally rotates the arm. The supraspinatus muscle is innervated by the suprascapular nerve C_4, C_5, C_6 (Fig. 17).

23

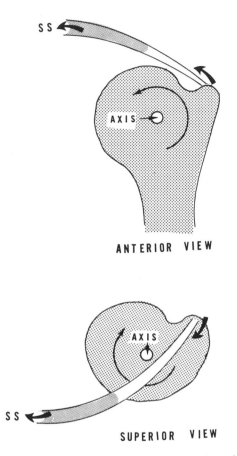

ANTERIOR VIEW

SUPERIOR VIEW

FIGURE 16. Function of supraspinatus muscle. Anterior view shows supraspinatus function abducting arm in the coronal plane. Viewed from superior view, this muscle externally rotates the arm.

The infraspinatus muscle originates from the greater surface area of the infraspinatus fossa of the scapula located below the spine of the scapula (see Fig. 15). The muscle proceeds laterally to insert just below the attachment of the supraspinatus muscle on the greater tuberosity. The tendons of the supraspinatus, the infraspinatus, and the teres minor merge into a conjoined tendon before attachment (see Fig. 13). The infraspinatus also passes superiorly and anteriorly to the axis of rotation but pulls in a slightly downward direction so it functions as does the supraspi-

24

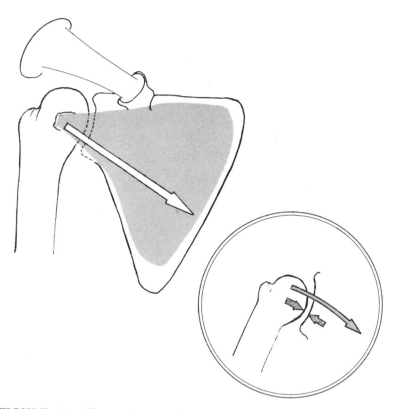

FIGURE 17. The subscapularis muscle. The subscapularis muscle originates from the entire anterior surface of the scapula, the surface that glides against the thoracic wall. The muscle extends laterally and attaches to the lesser tuberosity of the humerus. Its tendon is the most medial of those forming the "cuff." Its action is to pull the head of the humerus into the glenoid fossa and slightly downward.

natus plus causing the head of the humerus to glide down the glenoid fossa. The infraspinatus muscle is also innervated by the suprascapular nerve C_4, C_5, C_6.

The teres minor muscle arises from the lateral portion of the axillary border of the scapula (see Fig. 14) and passes laterally and upward to insert on the humerus immediately below the infraspinatus, on the greater tuberosity. The teres minor, originating lower on the scapula (see Fig. 14), also abducts and rotates the arm but more significantly depresses the head of the humerus.

25

The teres minor receives a branch of the axillary nerve as it proceeds to the deltoid muscle, C_5 and C_6.

The subscapularis muscle (Fig. 17) is the most anterior and the most medial muscle of the cuff. It originates from the entire anterior (thoracic) surface of the scapula and proceeds laterally to attach to the lesser tuberosity of the head of the humerus. The lesser tuberosity is located just medial to the bicipital groove. The subscapularis muscle passes in front of the shoulder joint and is separated from the neck of the scapula by a bursa. This bursa (see Fig. 8) is a pouching of the synovial cavity of the shoulder joint. By passing anterior to the axis of rotation, the subscapularis muscle is a powerful internal rotator of the arm. The muscle receives its nerve supply from the upper and lower subscapular nerves C_5 and C_6.[9]

There is an opening in the anterior portion of the cuff insertion upon the humerus, located between the supraspinatus muscle and the subscapularis muscle, through which the biceps tendon, its sheath, and an invagination of the synovial cavity pass. This opening is reinforced by the coracohumeral ligament, a ligament that proceeds from the coracoid process and fuses into the anterosuperior aspect of the glenohumeral capsule. There is further reinforcement by the transverse humeral ligament (see Fig. 8) that holds the biceps tendon in the biceps groove. The cuff's tendinous insertion is a conjoined tendon of all four cuff muscles: the supraspinatus, infraspinatus, teres minor, and subscapularis.

BURSAE

Bursae permit frictionless movement, but when inflamed may restrict glenohumeral joint motion. The subacromial bursa adheres at its inferior border to the greater tuberosity and the cuff. The roof adheres to the under surface of the acromium and the coracoacromial ligament (Fig. 18). The subscapular bursa is a prolongation of the synovial capsule. Intrabursal adhesions limit movement of the shoulder.

26

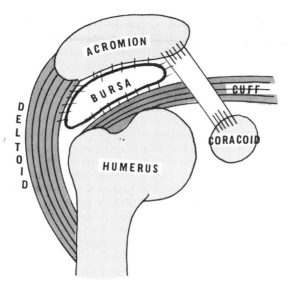

FIGURE 18.   Subacromial bursa.

NERVE SUPPLY TO SHOULDER

The articular branch of the circumflex (axillary) nerve C_5, C_6, as derived from the posterior cord, accompanies the posterior circumflex artery around the neck of the humerus. It has two divisions with the inferior branch being sensory and supplying the skin over the lower portion of the deltoid (Fig. 19). This branch is considered to be the only branch to the joint capsule.

The suprascapular nerve is considered by some not to be involved in sensation of the shoulder joint. Others disagree and feel that this is the innervation of the superior and posterior portion of the joint capsule and the greater part of the tendinous sheaths. The sensory fibers supply the acromioclavicular joint and the cuff portion of the shoulder.

All tissues of the shoulder girdle are supplied by somatic sensory nerves, i.e., tendons, bursae, ligaments, synovial tissues, capsule, and muscles. They produce *trigger points* that create tissue sites of pain.

There is a *critical zone* in the cuff that is the site of painful disabling pathology, for example, tendinitis, calcific deposits, or

27

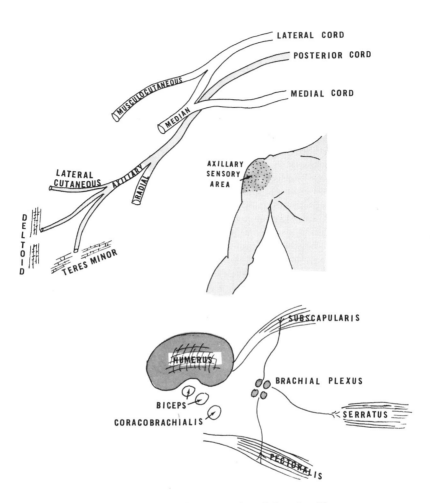

FIGURE 19. Nerve supply of the shoulder.

tear. This zone is the area of vascular anastomosis between the osseous arteries and the muscular arteries (Fig. 20). During passive dependence of the arm, this anastomosis is compressed making the zone ischemic. During active contraction of the cuff muscles during abduction or forward flexion, the cuff is also rendered ischemic. Only when the arm is in the resting and supported position is the zone hyperemic or at least adequately blood supplied (Fig. 21).

28

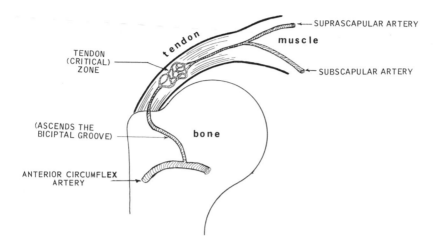

FIGURE 20. Circulation of the tendons of the cuff: the *critical zone*. The tendons of the cuff have a highly vascular zone at the anastomosis of the muscular vessels and the osseous vessels. This *critical zone* is the portion with the greatest tensile strength and is also the area that accumulates the calcium deposits; thus it is the site of cuff ruptures. This zone is graphically shown, and the contributing vessels are identified.

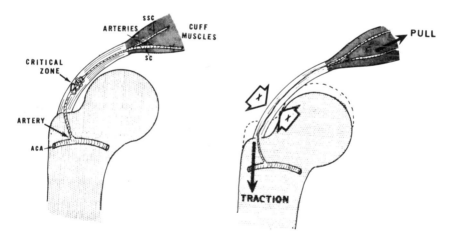

FIGURE 21. Blood circulation. *Left,* Circulation to the rotator cuff. The arterial branch from the anterior circumflex artery *(ACA)* enters from the bone. The suprascapular *(SSC)* and the subscapular *(SC)* branches merge to enter from the muscle. The critical zone of the tendon is an anastomosis which is patent when the arm is supported and inactive. *Right,* Traction upon the cuff from the dependent arm or from pull of the contracting cuff muscle elongates the tendon and renders the critical zone *(arrows)* relatively ischemic.

29

GLENOHUMERAL MOVEMENT

In the passive dangling arm, the stability of the glenohumeral joint is now clearly understood not to be muscular. The joint is stable and downward dislocation is prevented by the angulation of the glenoid fossa and the mechanical support of the superior portion of the capsule and supraspinatus muscle. Both the capsule and supraspinatus muscle are horizontally aligned and prevent the head of the humerus from gliding down the glenoid fossa. With the glenoid fossa angled facing forward, outward, and upward as the humerus slides downward, the capsule and cuff mechanically become more taut. This prevents further descent (Fig. 22).

Bringing the humerus in any degree of abduction or forward flexion eliminates this support and places the stability upon mus-

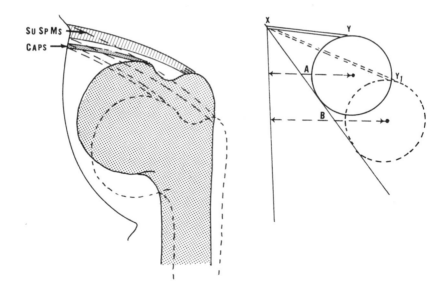

FIGURE 22. Capsular-passive cuff support. Due to the orientation of the glenoid fossa which faces forward, outward, and upward, the superior capsule, being taut in the normal position, becomes more taut as the humeral head (A) descends. B depicts an analogy of a ball rolling down an angled plane.

30

cular contraction. Depression of the glenoid fossa as a result of downward rotation of the scapula causes adduction of the arm and, therefore, requires muscular effort to support the arm. This may well be a significant factor in the subluxation and painful dysfunction of the hemiplegic shoulder.

Abduction of the arm in the coronal plane (Fig. 23) is possible only by downward gliding of the head of the humerus to allow the greater tuberosity to pass under the overhanging acromion and coracoacromial arch. This complex movement occurs by coordinated action of the cuff muscles and the deltoid muscle or what has become known as the *scapulohumeral rhythm*.

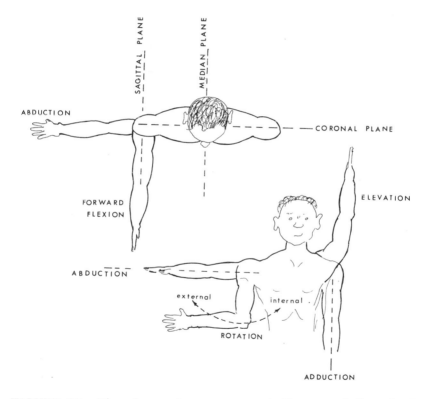

FIGURE 23. The planes of arm movement. Terms used throughout the text state the direction of movement and the planes of movement in relationship to the body. The body is viewed from above and from the front. All arm planes are related to these two body positions.

The *deltoid muscle* (Fig. 24) arises anteriorly from the clavicle, laterally from the acromion, and posteriorly from the spine of the scapula, and passes down in front of, lateral to, and behind the shoulder glenohumeral joint. The fibers attach to the anterior lateral area of the middle third of the humerus. The basic action of deltoid contraction is elevation of the humerus along a line parallel to the humerus and tends to force the humeral head up against the coracoacromial ligament. When working in harmony with the cuff muscles, the middle (lateral) fibers of the deltoid abduct the arm in the coronal plane. The anterior deltoid fibers forward flex in the sagittal plane while slightly internally rotating

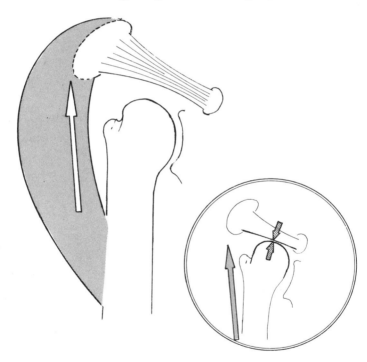

FIGURE 24. Deltoid muscle and its isolated function. The deltoid muscle originates from the inferior aspect of the spine of the scapula and the protruding acromial process. By its attachment into the humeral shaft, it has a direction of pull as depicted by the arrow in the large figure. Its isolated action shown in the circle is that of elevation, impinging the head of the humerus directly up under the coracoacromial arch. As the head of the humerus is rotated, depressed, and adducted into the glenoid fossa by the other cuff muscles, the deltoid becomes a powerful *ab*ductor.

the humerus. The posterior fibers extend the humerus posteriorly in the sagittal plane and externally rotate the humerus. The deltoid muscle is innervated by the axillary nerve (C_5 and C_6).

The deltoid muscle with its origin from the acromial process and its insertion into the lateral aspect of the upper one third of the humerus exerts its line of pull along the shaft of the humerus. Its primary action is to elevate the humerus, thus abutting the head of the humerus up against the coracohumeral head. With slight abduction of the humerus performed by the cuff muscles, the deltoid has an angular pull upon the humerus to now make it an abductor rather than an elevator (Fig. 25).

To permit abduction of the arm, the head of the humerus must be rotated within the glenoid fossa and the articulating

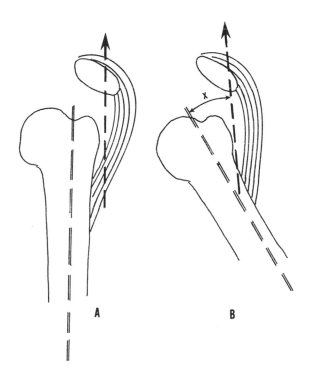

FIGURE 25. Abduction angle of deltoid. *A*, With the arm dependent, the deltoid line of pull is along the line of the humerus and thus elevates the arm up against the acromion. *B*, With slight abduction of the humerus the angle of the deltoid changes its pull to abduction of the arm.

surface of the humerus made to glide downward and be *fixed* against the fossa for stability. This motion is performed by the cuff muscles to permit the greater tuberosity to pass under the coracoacromial cuff and to change the angle of insertion of the deltoid to make the muscle an abductor (Fig. 25).

Analysis of the action of the cuff reveals that the *supraspinatus* originates from the supraspinatus fossa of the scapula and passes horizontally under the coracoacromial head to insert upon the greater tuberosity of the humerus. By passing slightly superior to the axis of rotation of the humeral head, it exerts some rotation of the head to cause some degree of rotation. Its horizontal alignment seats the head of the humerus into the glenoid fossa. This latter action is probably its major function.[9] Early studies of kinesiology asserted that the supraspinatus muscle initiated and acted during the first degrees of abduction with its maximum activity at 100° of abduction. Recent electromyographic studies[10] have disproven this and shown that the supraspinatus is active throughout the entire abduction of the arm in the coronal plane. Supraspinatus paralysis merely diminishes the strength and endurance of abduction of the arm but has no influence upon the range of motion.[11]

The *infraspinatus* originating from the infraspinatus fossa attaches after a horizontal route into the tuberosity. Its action is also to seat the head of the humerus and cause some rotation but it also pulls the head down the glenoid fossa. The *teres minor* by its angulation between origin and insertion depresses the humeral head into the glenoid fossa. The subscapularis also lowers the humeral head as well as fixing it into the glenoid fossa. Therefore, the combined action of the cuff muscles is to (1) rotate the humerus in the coronal plane into abduction, (2) seat the head into the glenoid fossa for stability, and (3) glide the humeral head downward in the glenoid fossa (Fig. 26). All these actions assist the deltoid to become an *abductor*.

The cuff muscles also rotate the humerus about its longitudinal axis in internal and external rotation of the arm. This function is mandatory to assure proper abduction and elevation of the arm

34

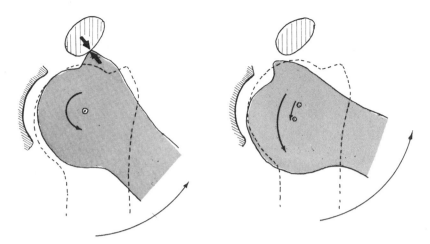

FIGURE 26. Glenohumeral movement of arm abduction. The incongruity of the articular surface of the head of the humerus and the surface of the glenoid fossa is shown. *Left*. The greater tuberosity of the humerus impinging upon the coracoacromial ligament if rotation is not accompanied by depression of the humerus. *Right*, Simultaneous depression and rotation in a *gliding* motion permitting the greater tuberosity to pass under the coracoacromial hood during arm abduction.

and will be subsequently discussed (Fig. 27). Abduction of the arm is possible only with simultaneous rotation of the humerus which permits the greater tuberosity of the humerus to pass posteriorly to the acromial process. With the humerus in internal rotation, only 60° of abduction is possible due to the fact that the humerus, in internal rotation, impinges much earlier upon the coracoacromial ligament than it does in external rotation (Fig. 28).

To permit the arm to abduct and elevate fully overhead (an arc of 180°), an additional 60° must combine with the active 90° and passive 120° occurring at the glenohumeral joint. This motion results from rotation of the scapula which adds an additional 60° to overhead elevation of the arm. The combined movement of the humerus upon the scapula at the glenohumeral joint and the scapula upon the thorax, in its simultaneous synchronous movement, conforms to the well established *Codman scapulohumeral rhythm.*[12]

Forward flexion of the shoulder is achieved by (1) the cla-

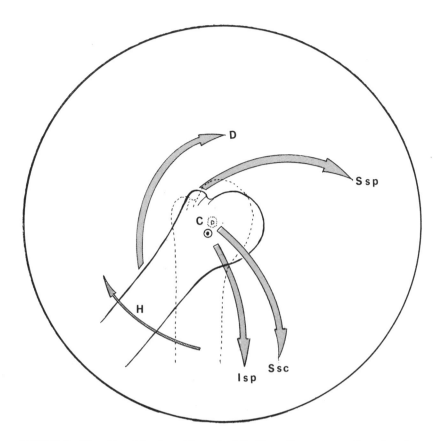

FIGURE 27. Combined cuff and deltoid action upon the glenohumeral articulation. Abduction of the humerus along the plane *H* is the result of combined action of the supraspinatus, *Ssp,* adducting the head into the fossa; the infraspinatus and subscapularis, *Isp* and *Ssc,* adducting and depressing the head; and the deltoid, *D,* acting as an abductor when working with these cuff muscles. The center of rotation, *C,* lowers during this downward gliding motion.

vicular head of the pectoralis major, (2) the anterior fibers of deltoid, and (3) both heads of the bicep. Before discussing this total arm movement, the scapular phase of the rhythm requires evaluation.

SCAPULAR MOVEMENT

The scapula moves in a gliding manner upon the thoracic wall at the thoracoscapular articulation. Movement occurs at the distal

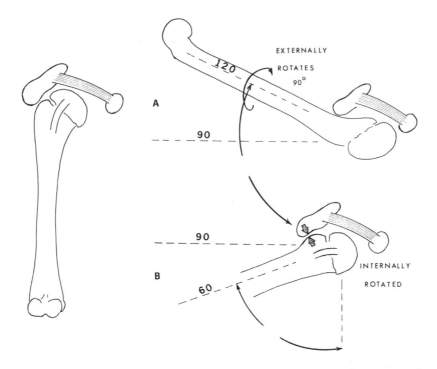

FIGURE 28. Influence of humeral rotation upon abduction range of the glenohumeral joint. *A,* Active abduction is possible to 90°, and an additional 30° can be gained passively if the humerus rotates externally approximately through a 90° arc. This abduction range of 120° is possible because the rotation allows the greater tuberosity to pass behind the acromion. *B,* With the arm internally rotated, the greater tuberosity impinges against the coracoacromial arch and blocks abduction at 60°.

end of the clavicle, the acromioclavicular joint, by virtue of motion and rotation of the clavicle. Motion of the scapula is primarily produced by two muscles, the trapezius and the serratus anterior.

The broad fan-shaped trapezius muscle acts as three muscles (Fig. 29). The upper fibers of the trapezius originate from the ligamentum nuchae in the lower cervical region, the posterior spinous processes of the cervical spine, and the upper thoracic spine. They radiate laterally and downward to attach to the upper margin of the medial and central portion of the scapular spine. The action of the upper trapezius pulls the scapula upward and causes inward pivoting about the acromioclavicular joint.

37

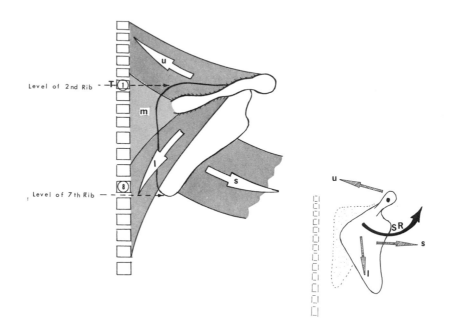

FIGURE 29. Scapular musculature: Rotators. The scapular muscles forming the rotator phase of the *scapulohumeral rhythm* are shown with the upper trapezius fibers elevating the outer border of the spine, the lower fibers of the trapezius depressing the medial border of the spine, and the serratus pulling the lower portion of the scapula forward from its position under the blade. The combined action moves the scapula in orbit around the acromioclavicular center of rotation.

u = upper		s = serratus anterior
m = middle } trapezius		SR = scapular rotation
l = lower		

The middle fibers originate from the spinous processes of the upper thoracic vertebrae, proceed laterally, and attach to the medial border of the scapular spine. These middle fibers principally "fix" the scapula during abduction of the arm. They must relax during forward flexion of the arm-shoulder in the sagittal plane.

The lower fibers of the trapezius originate from the spinous processes of the lower thoracic vertebrae and attach to the medial portion of the spine of the scapula. The isolated function of these fibers pulls the medial border of the spine of the scapula *down*

38

and *in*. The combined action of the upper and lower trapezius fibers rotates the scapula around the axis center of the acromioclavicular joint, depressing the vertebral border, and elevating the glenoid fossa on the outer portion. The trapezius is supplied by the spinal accessory nerve (XI.).

The serratus anterior is the other major muscle acting to rotate the scapula. This broad muscle originates from the upper eight ribs of the anterolateral chest wall, anterior to the scapula, and runs posteriorly to insert upon the medial (vertebral) border of the scapula. The heaviest fibers attach upon the inferior border. The serratus is located in the *scapulocostal joint* space between the scapula and the rib cage. Its line of pull moves the scapula forward and, because it acts below the axis of the acromioclavicular joint, acts as a rotator. The serratus muscle is innervated by the long thoracic nerve formed by the anterior branches of the roots of C_5, C_6, and C_7 (primarily C_6) before they enter the brachial plexus.

The combined action of the upper trapezius, the lower trapezius, and the serratus causes rotation of the scapula about the pivotal point of the acromioclavicular joint and elevates the glenoid fossa.

There are other muscles that act upon the scapula but are not involved in the scapulohumeral rhythm. Under the trapezius are three muscles that attach to the vertebral border of the scapula: the levator scapula, the rhomboid major, and the rhomboid minor (Fig. 30). The levator scapula originates from the cervical transverse processes and proceeds downward and laterally to attach to the superior angle of the scapula. The rhomboid minor is located immediately below the levator, originates from the lower cervical vertebra, and attaches to the vertebral border of the scapula at the level of the scapular spine. The rhomboid major, much broader than the above muscles, originates from the upper thoracic vertebrae and inserts into the remainder of the vertebral border of the scapula. They elevate the medial aspect of the scapula and cause downward rotation of the glenoid fossa by

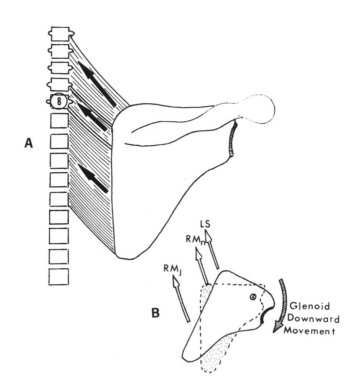

FIGURE 30. Downward rotators of the scapula. The muscles acting upon the scapula directly to cause downward rotation of the glenoid fossa are the levator scapulae (upper arrow), the rhomboid minor (middle arrow), and the rhomboid major (lower arrow).

virtue of the rotation around the acromioclavicular pivotal point. These three muscles receive their nerve supply from C_5 through the dorsal scapular nerve.

The pectoralis major and latissimus dorsi also act upon the scapula by virtue of their attachment upon the humerus. These muscles, as well as the levator scapulae and rhomboids, all are involved in the hemiplegic shoulder by their imbalance, spasticity, and incoordination, and merit a great deal of attention.

The *pectoralis major* is a large thick muscle attached upon the anterior chest wall running from the clavicle, sternum, and ribs as three bands (Fig. 31). Both the clavicular and the manubrial fibers run straight from origin to insertion and are most superficial. The deep fibers from the sternum and ribs twist in their

40

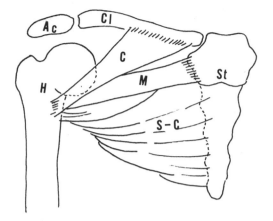

FIGURE 31. Pectoralis major. The pectoralis major has three laminae: clavicular (C), manubrial (M), and a sternocostal (S-C) bundle. All form the pectoralis muscle but are considered to have slightly separate functions (see text).

course to the humerus. The clavicular portion, by its direction, acts to flex the humerus. The manubrial fibers horizontally adduct and internally rotate the arm. When the arm is hyperextended (posteriorly flexed) these fibers assist in forward flexion of the arm. The pectoralis major muscle is innervated by the two anterior thoracic nerves with roots of the last four cervical and first thoracic (T_1) nerve. The clavicular portion receives innervation from C_5–C_6 the sternal portion from C_7–C_8 and T_1.

The *latissimus dorsi* is a large posterior muscle that originates from the iliac crest and the spines of all the lumbar and the lower six thoracic vertebrae. The fibers converge upward and laterally to curve around the medial aspect of the humerus to the medial lip of the bicipital groove. The chief function of the latissimus dorsi is that of adduction, extension, and internal rotation of the arm and depression of the shoulder girdle. The latissimus dorsi is more influential for internal rotation than is the pectoralis major which only shows internal rotation when resisted.

The *pectoralis minor* is a relatively small muscle that originates from the outer surfaces of ribs 3, 4, and 5 and passes upward and laterally to attach to the coracoid process. In contraction, this

41

muscle causes abduction and downward rotation of the scapula. In this action, it pulls the vertebral border of the scapula away from the ribs and also changes the angulation of the glenoid fossa. Its function in hemiplegia is not clear.

SCAPULOHUMERAL MOVEMENT

Abduction elevation of the arm in the coronal plane, from dependency at the side of the body until fully extended overhead, with palms facing each other, is a smooth, synchronous motion involving every component of the shoulder girdle complex. Motion must be smooth and effortless, requiring full range of motion at each joint and well-coordinated muscle balance. *The normal composite movement is stressed because knowledge and recognition of the slightest imbalance and restriction must be recognized to evaluate* the abnormal patterns of the spastic and flacid hemiplegic shoulder.

The smooth, integrated movement of the humerus, the scapula, and the clavicle has been well termed the "scapulohumeral rhythm" by Dr. E. A. Codman, whose book, *The shoulder,* is monumental (Fig. 32).[12]

Of every 15° of abduction of the arm, 10° occur at the glenohumeral joint, and 5° from rotation of the scapula upon the chest wall. This 2:1 ratio of humerus to scapula exists throughout the entire abduction range in a smooth, rhythmic pattern. To reiterate, the scapula can rotate 60°; the humerus, 90° actively and 120° passively.

The scapula rotates to maintain mechanical stability of the glenohumeral joint and efficiency of the deltoid muscle. The deltoid, as all muscles, has greatest efficiency at its *rest length,* the point midway between its extremes of motion. The deltoid is at rest length when the arm is dependent at the side. Abduction shortens the muscle, and by 90° abduction with no scapular rotation, the extreme of contraction is reached. The deltoid then is barely able to support the arm. Scapular rotation maintains optimum deltoid length throughout abduction (Fig. 33).

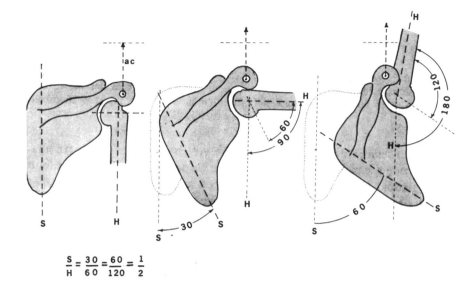

$$\frac{S}{H} = \frac{30}{60} = \frac{60}{120} = \frac{1}{2}$$

FIGURE 32. Scapulohumeral rhythm (Codman). The scapula and the humerus at position of rest with the scapula relaxed and the arm dependent, both at position 0°. The abduction movement of the arm is accomplished in a smooth, coordinated movement during which for each 15° of arm abduction 10° of motion occur at the glenohumeral joint and 5° occur due to scapular rotation upon the thorax. The humerus, *H*, has abducted 90° in relationship to the erect body, but this has been accomplished by 30° rotation of the scapula and 60° of the humerus at the glenohumeral joint: 2:1 ratio. *Right,* Full elevation of the arm: 60° at the scapula and 120° at the glenohumeral joint.

Full overhead elevation requires little or no deltoid support if the scapula has fully rotated. At this point the glenoid fossa is directly under the head of the humerus. Had there been no scapular rotation, the humerus could not fully abduct or elevate overhead (see Fig. 32).

In hemiparesis, the muscles that permit this scapulohumeral rhythm are impaired by overwhelming spasticity of the antagonist and the abductor. External rotation and elevation of the arm is prevented. Scapulohumeral movement of the glenohumeral joint and the scapulothoracic joint has been highlighted with "motion around the axis of the acromioclavicular joint." This joint and the sternoclavicular joint play a vital role in the total arm motion.

43

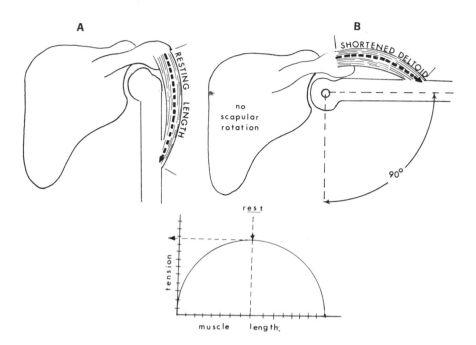

FIGURE 33. Deltoid action upon the glenohumeral joint. The mechanical efficiency afforded the deltoid action upon abduction of the humerus by the simultaneous rotation of the scapula is shown in the length-tension relationship upon muscle. Muscle efficiency is greatest at *rest* length and diminishes upon shortening. In the abducted arm without scapular rotation, the deltoid shortens to a length of less tension. (*B*). Simultaneous scapular rotation keeps the deltoid at *rest* length (*A*).

ACROMIOCLAVICULAR AND STERNOCLAVICULAR JOINTS

The acromioclavicular joint is a plane joint connecting the outer end of the clavicle with its convex facet to the anterior medial portion of the acromial process. A fibrocartilaginous ring that resembles an intra-articular meniscus may exist.

The clavicle is firmly attached to the scapula by the coracoclavicular ligament. Two resilient fascicles, each called a ligament, form the coracoclavicular ligament: the lateral *trapezoid* and the medial *conoid* ligaments. The manner of attachment of these ligaments prevents the scapula from rotating about the acromiocla-

44

vicular joint and, by its "strut" shape, maintains a constant relationship of the scapula to the clavicle (Fig. 34).

The coracoclavicular ligament, by its attachments in a strut shape, was once considered instrumental in holding the scapula away from the chest wall and giving stability to the acromioclavicular joint. This is now disproven by the retention of stability after severence of this ligament. Instability results *only* when there is severence of the coracoclavicular ligament *and* the superior acromioclavicular ligament.

As the scapula rotates to elevate the glenoid fossa, it rotates the clavicle about its long axis through the attachment of the coracoclavicular ligaments to the outer end of the clavicle. The "crank" shape of the clavicle elevates the outer end with no change in the angle of elevation at the proximal sternoclavicular joint. Rotation of the clavicle occurs primarily in the overhead

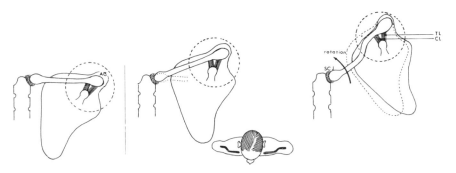

FIGURE 34.   Action of the coracoclavicular ligaments upon the acromioclavicular joint. The coracoclavicular ligament attaches the scapula to the clavicle. It is divided into two resilient fascicles termed the *trapezoid* ligament and the *conoid* ligament. From the coracoid they proceed upward and laterally to attach onto the undersurface of the clavicle. Elevation of the clavicle without rotation maintains a constant relationship of the scapula to the clavicle. The rotation of the scapula depresses the coracoid and thus rotates the clavicle about its long axis.

The left drawing depicts the scapula at rest with the coracoclavicular ligaments viewed from (through) the sagittal axis (large dotted circle). The middle drawing shows abduction of the clavicle along the coronal plane without rotation. The right picture shows full elevation of the clavicle, still showing an unchanged relationship of the scapula to the clavicle in this coronal plane. Motion through this range must occur at the sternoclavicular joint, *SCJ*.

arm elevation above 90° abduction of the arm (Fig. 35). The first 30° of clavicular elevation occurs at the sternoclavicular joint. The next 30° of elevation is the result of rotation of the clavicle about its long axis.

The sternoclavicular joint is formed by the sternal end of the clavicle attaching to the superior lateral portion of the manubrium of the sternum and the cartilage of the first rib (Fig. 36). An articular disk between the sternum and the clavicle forms two joint spaces. Anterior and posterior sternoclavicular ligaments reinforce a loose fibrous capsule, and an interclavicular ligament connects the two clavicles. Stability of the joint is imparted by the costoclavicular ligament, a strong ligament that arises from the medial portion of the first rib and runs oblique laterally to

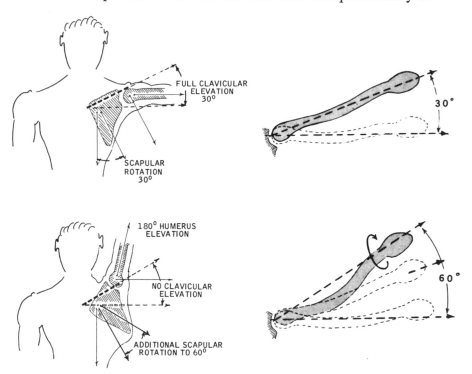

FIGURE 35. Scapular elevation resulting from clavicular rotation. The upper drawing shows the elevation of the clavicle without rotation to 30°. The remaining 30° of scapular rotation, which is imperative in full scapulohumeral range, occurs by rotation of the "crankshaped" clavicle about its long axis.

46

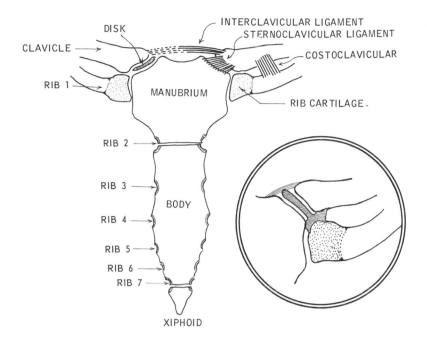

FIGURE 36. Sternoclavicular joint. The sternoclavicular joint is formed by the medial portion of the clavicle articulating upon the manubrium sterni and also with the cartilage end of the first rib. The ligaments that stabilize the joint are shown. The fibroelastic disk, or meniscus, is shown in the insert. In spite of marked movement at this joint in all shoulder girdle movements, arthritic changes are rare, mild, and rarely disabling.

attach into the undersurface of the clavicle. This ligament stabilizes the clavicle against muscle action (Fig. 37) and acts as a fulcrum for all motions of the shoulder girdle.

The sternoclavicular joint, in spite of its plane joint surfaces, acts like a ball-and-socket joint, participating in all motions of the shoulder complex. In spite of its excess use, unlike the acromioclavicular joint, degenerative changes occur late in life and are mild with minimal functional impediment.

COMPOSITE SHOULDER GIRDLE MOVEMENTS

Movement of the shoulder girdle requires smooth, effortless, synchronous movement of the glenohumeral joint and all the ac-

47

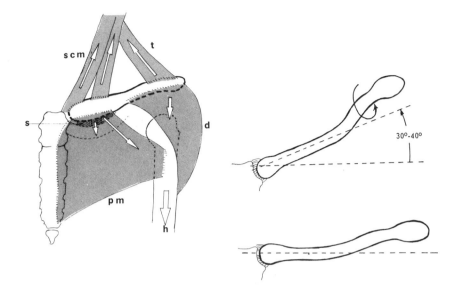

FIGURE 37. Muscles acting upon the clavicle. The major muscles acting upon the clavicle are shown, their direction of pull indicated by arrows: *scm*, sternocleidomastoid; *t*, trapezius; *d*, deltoid; *s*, subscapularis; and *pm*, pectoralis major. The gravity pull of the arm itself is represented by *h*. The muscles that act indirectly upon the clavicle are not shown.

cessory joints. Each has been individually considered; now the composite movement can be related.

When the arm is raised in abduction, the humerus and the scapula move in a rhythm so that for every 15° of total abduction of the arm 10° occur at the glenohumeral joint, with a corresponding 5° of rotation of the scapula. The humerus will complete its full possible abduction only if it externally rotates during elevation to permit the greater tuberosity to pass under and behind the coracoacromial ligament. Only 60° of humeral abduction is possible with the arm internally rotated. Only in the externally rotated position can the humerus abduct actively to 90°, and be passively abducted to 120°. Combined muscular action of the rotators and abductors performs this task.

Full elevation of the arm overhead (180°) requires 60° of scapular rotation to alter the angle of the glenoid fossa upon which the humerus articulates. Scapular rotation results from the combined action of the trapezius and serratus muscles. Because the coracoclavicular ligaments prevent scapular rotation in the coronal plane, the scapula pivots about the acromioclavicular joint from rotation of the crank-shaped clavicle and elevation at the sternoclavicular joint (see Fig. 35).

Motion of the sternoclavicular joint is possible in all planes. The clavicle and the scapula are elevated by the trapezius and other accessory muscles that attach to the clavicle. For every 10° of arm elevation, 4° of the elevation occurs at the clavicle. There is varying elevation of the clavicle during the total arm elevation phase. Approximately 15° of clavicular elevation occurs during the first 30° of arm abduction, and the clavicle has elevated to its final position as the arm reaches the horizontal level (90° abduction).

Half of the scapular rotation thus has been reached (30°) by clavicular elevation. The remaining 30° occurs by rotation of the crank-shaped clavicle exerting pull on the coracoid process through the coracoclavicular ligaments. The clavicle rotates 45°, which raises the clavicle and its attached scapula an additional 30°. The greater part, if not all the rotation, occurs in the arm elevation above the horizontal position.

With such an intricate synchronized neuromuscular mechanism, it is not surprising that voluntary restoration of function is so difficult to regain after hemiplegia or hemiparesis (Fig. 38).

BICEPS MECHANISM

The biceps is anatomically and pathologically involved in the shoulder girdle, but its kinetics is only indirectly related to glenohumeral movement. Beevor, in his coordination studies of the muscles of the shoulder, included the biceps (long head) in abduction of the arm and forward flexion as well as movement of the elbow (Fig. 39).

The biceps brachii has two heads but a common tendon insertion into the tuberosity upon the inner aspect of the radius.

49

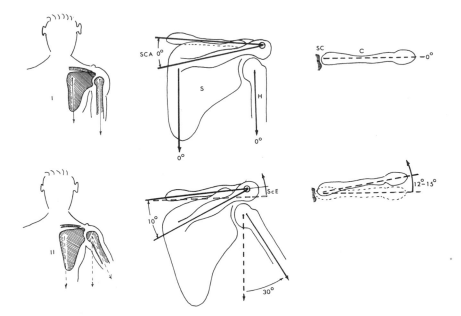

FIGURE 38. Accessory movement of the scapulohumeral rhythm other than the glenohumeral movement. Movement of the arm through all phases of abduction involves all joints of the shoulder girdle in a synchronous manner.

Phase I: The resting arm: 0° scapular rotation, *S;* 0° spinoclavicular angle, *SCA;* 0° movement at the sternoclavicular joint, *SC;* no elevation of the outer end of the clavicle, *C;* no abduction of the humerus, *H.*

Phase II: Humerus abducted 30°: outer end of clavicle elevated 12° to 15° with no rotation of the clavicle; elevation occurs at the sterno-clavicular joint; some movement occurs at the acromioclavicular joint as seen by increase of 10° of the spinoclavicular angle (*angle formed by the clavicle and the scapular spine*).

The short medial head originates from the coracoid process. The long head originates from the superior lip of the glenoid fossa, proceeds laterally, and angles 90° at the bicipital groove of the humerus, to proceed downward to the common tendon.

By its attachment on the ulnar side of the radius, its action is primarily supination of the forearm and secondarily elbow flex-

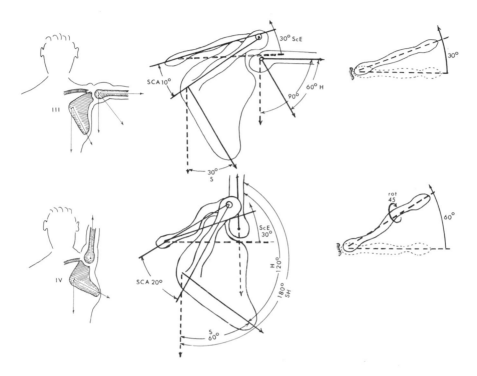

Phase III: Humerus, *H,* abducted to 90° (60° glenohumeral, 30° scapular): clavicle elevated to its final position, 30°; no rotation of clavicle as yet—all movement at the sternoclavicular joint; no change in the *SCA.*

Phase IV: Full overhead elevation (*SH* 180°–*H* 120°–*S* 60°): outer end of clavicle has not elevated further (at the sternoclavicular joint), but the *SCA* has increased (to 20°). Because of the clavicle's rotation and its "cranklike" form, the clavicle elevates an additional 30°. The humerus through this phase has rotated, but this has not influenced the above degrees of movement.

ion. In the upper arm region the biceps assists the anterior deltoid in forward flexing the shoulder.

In abducting the arm, the biceps groove glides along the long biceps tendon. The biceps tendon in essence *does not* glide along the groove. After 90° abduction, the tendon would leave the groove were it not for the transverse humeral ligament (Fig. 9). With abduction and rotation of the humerus, the tendon assumes an angle that has the tendency to sublux it from the groove.

51

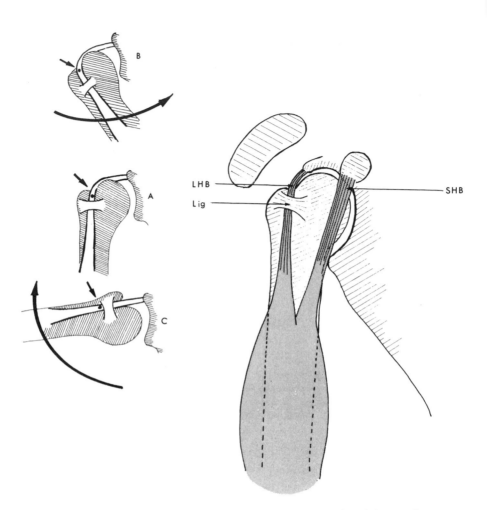

FIGURE 39. Biceps mechanism. The biceps brachii originates from two tendons: the short medial head, from the coracoid process; and the long head, from the superior rim of the glenoid fossa. The long head passes down into the bicipital groove in a fibrous sheath between the tendons of the subscapularis and the supraspinatus tendon. The small figures depict the movement of the humerus *upon* the biceps tendon. *A,* The dependent hanging arm. *B,* Arm adducted, internally rotated, and extended, causing the ligament (*dot*) to move away from the transverse humeral ligament. *C,* depicts downward movement of the ligament (*dot*) below the transverse humeral ligament when the arm is abducted, externally rotated, and flexed forward.

52

SUMMARY

Much space has been devoted to the functional anatomy of the shoulder. Without this knowledge, a meaningful clinical examination cannot be performed. In the hemiplegic patient as in the nonhemiplegic, pain and impairment cannot be established without a careful evaluation of every aspect of this intricate mechanism.

A clear and precise evaluation of faulty neuromuscular action combined with the ascertaining of free full passive range of motion is mandatory to understand the hemiplegic shoulder. This fundamental knowledge and observation can lead to a constructive treatment program.[13]

REFERENCES

1. DePalma, A. F.: Surgery of the Shoulder. J. B. Lippincott Co., Philadelphia, 1950.
2. Moseley, H. F. and Overgaard, B.: Anterior capsular mechanism in recurrent anterior dislocation of shoulder: Morphological and clinical studies with special reference to Glenoid labrum and glenohumeral ligament. J. Bone Joint Surg. 44–B:913, 1962.
3. Kleinberg, S.: Lesions of the musculotendenous cuff of the shoulder. J. Bone Joint Surg. 26:50, 1944.
4. Rowe, C. R., and Sakellarides, H. T.: Factors related to recurrent dislocation of the shoulder. Clin. Orthop. 20:40, 1961.
5. Inman, V. E., Saunders, J. B., and Abbott, L. C.: Observations in the function of the shoulder joint. J. Bone Joint Surg. 26:1, 1944.
6. Moseley, H. F.: Shoulder Lesions, ed. 3. Churchill Livingstone, New York, 1969, pp. 1–21, 60–68.
7. Steindler, A.: Lectures on the Interpretation of Pain in Orthopedic Practice. Charles C Thomas, Springfield, Ill, 1959.
8. Haymaker, W. and Woodhall, B.: Peripheral Nerve Injuries, W. B. Saunders Co., Philadelphia, 1953.
9. Hall, M. C.: The Locomotor System: Functional Anatomy. Charles C Thomas, Springfield, Ill, 1965, pp. 206–232.
10. Basmajion, J. V.: Muscles Alive. William & Wilkins Co., Baltimore, 1974.
11. VanLinge, B. and Mulder J. D.: The function of the supraspinous muscle and its relation to the supraspinous syndrome. J. Bone Joint Surg. 45 B:750, 1963.
12. Codman, E. A.: The Shoulder. Thomas Todd Co., Boston, 1934.
13. Cailliet, R.: Shoulder Pain. F. A. Davis Co., Philadelphia, 1966.

CHAPTER 3

Flaccid Stage

FLAIL EXTREMITY

In the early phase of hemiplegia, the patient develops flail extremities on the hemiplegic side. He loses "contact" with the involved limb so that he cannot feel the extremity and cannot move it. The limb can be passively moved in full range of motion and no resistance is encountered. No spasticity exists. Although the unaffected side should be expected to function, it does not compensate for the loss of function of the affected side. The patient usually assumes lateral flexion of the head toward the affected side, and the trunk also laterally flexes toward that side. Sitting balance is not possible or is at best precarious. The hand and fingers assume a flexed position and the shoulder girdle becomes retracted and depressed. With return of any tone in the arm, the elbow assumes a flexed position with the forearm pronated. The flaccid status occurs because the excitatory center of the spinal cord is depressed or actually absent. There is no internuncial pool activity. Upon attempting any active movement of the unaffected side, there are usually no associated movements of the affected side. During the flaccid stage, positioning of the patient to prevent secondary tissue damage is indicated. Training to restore volitional motor response begins with sensory stimulation to initiate reflex activity. The numerous techniques of initiating reflex activity include:

1. Stretch reflex (via muscle spindles)
2. Tapping of the tendon
3. Vibration: manual or mechanical
4. Brushing or stroking to elicit cutaneous flexion response
5. Cooling of the skin by ice or vasocoolant spray
6. Tonic neck reflexes
7. Labyrinthine reflexes
8. Reflex synergies

Sensory feedback is essential to reestablish specific patterns of movement and coordination. This sensory feedback may occur from joint proprioception, visual observation, muscular activity, auditory confirmation by the therapist, or cutaneous stimulation. Currently, biofeedback reeducation by electromyography is enjoying enthusiastic exploration.

Rotation of the head and neck towards or away from the involved side can initiate either a flexor or extensor pattern of the upper or lower extremity. Usually turning the head toward the uninvolved side causes flexion, abduction, and external rotation of the involved shoulder.[1] Neck flexion usually initiates flexor patterns of the upper extremity. These tonic neck reflexes are limited to the first three cervical nerves (Magnus and de Kleijn).[1] McCoach showed that these tonic neck reflexes remained after sectioning all muscular and cutaneous branches of C_1, C_2, C_3 but disappeared upon sectioning the capsular nerve branch of the upper three cervical vertebrae. As no pattern is predictably specific, various positions of the head and neck must be tried to acquire the desired pattern (Fig. 40).[1,2]

The body responds to labyrinthine reflexes and these can be used to enhance reflex activity in the involved extremities. Insofar as body relationship to gravity influences the arm-shoulder reflexes, the supine position encourages flexor tone in the upper extremity examination. Position of the patient during treatment must bear this in mind. Frequently, side lying or sitting is a more favorable position to evaluate and treat the patient rather than the usually used supine position. Whereas in the supine position,

56

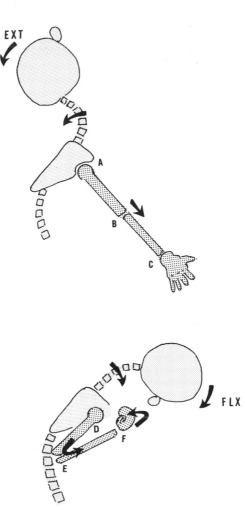

FIGURE 40. Upper illustration depicts the extensor pattern of the upper extremity in neck extension. The lower drawing shows flexion of the upper extremity on neck flexion. *A*, shoulder; *B*, elbow; *C*, wrist; *E*, elbow flexed; *F*, wrist-fingers flexed.

the lower extremities tend to extend at the hip with external rotation of the leg, when there is return of reflexes in the upper extremity, the shoulder usually retracts posteriorly with internal rotation and flexion of the elbow, wrist, and fingers. The latissimus dorsi muscle functions to retract the shoulder and internally rotate the arm as well as laterally flex the trunk, therefore,

57

this muscle must be carefully observed for its involvement in affecting this position.

Treatment

Considering the position of the flail extremity and its relationship to gravity and total body position, proper positioning must be utilized to neutralize undesirable positions of the arm.

1. The supine position must be avoided or at least minimized. Ultimately, if flaccidity proceeds to spasticity, which it usually does, extension and retraction of the arm in the spastic phase will be enforced by the supine position.
2. The patient must be assisted to lie on his side, either on the affected or unaffected arm, with the shoulder in a slightly forward flexed position with the elbow extended. This position can be maintained by properly placed pillows or more easily by the ingenious use of the air inflated splint advocated by Johnstone (Fig. 41).[3]
3. The patient's head should be flexed laterally and rotated toward the unaffected side.
4. The trunk should be laterally flexed away from the affected side.

It is permissible and, in fact, desirable to have the patient lie on the involved side with the arm flexed well forward at the shoulder, the elbow extended, and the forearm supinated.

Before any active rehabilitation exercises are begun for the extremities, trunk movements must be initiated. Rolling over to either side should be started. As trunk or neck movements may initiate extremity spastic patterns, undesirable positions of the upper extremity should be guarded against. The following positions should be avoided:

1. Retraction (posterior flexion) of the shoulder
2. Depression of the shoulder girdle

58

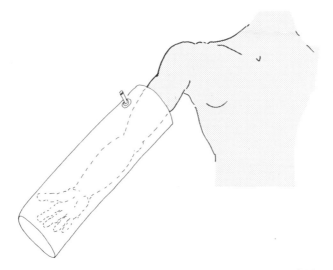

FIGURE 41. The entire upper extremity is enclosed within an air-inflated splint. The warmth of the breath that inflates the splint and the complete skin contact supposedly act as reflex stimulators. The elbow is extended as are the wrist and fingers, and the entire arm can be placed in abduction and external rotation. Thus the shoulder can be positioned and exercised.

3. Adduction of the arm
4. Internal rotation of the arm
5. Elbow flexion
6. Pronation of the forearm
7. Ulnar deviation of the wrist
8. Flexion of the wrist and fingers
9. Adduction of the thumb

As the patient gradually learns to move from the supine position to the prone position, the arm is held flexed forward at the shoulder with the elbow extended. In the supine position, the arm is supinated at the forearm, extended at the wrist and elbow, thumb abducted, and the arm is gradually raised to the overhead position maintaining full extension and external rotation (Fig. 42). Throughout all passive movements of the extremity, the patient is asked to *try* to hold the arm in various positions along

59

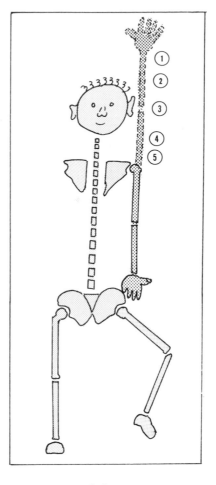

(Y)

FIGURE 42. With patient supine, the extremity is gradually raised to the overhead position: 1 and 2, the forearm is supinated; 3, the elbow extended; 4, abducted; 5, the upper arm externally rotated.

the course of movement. This encourages active control of the extremity (Fig. 43).

The glenohumeral joint should be mobilized manually by the therapist to ensure that the humerus does not depress or retract. The therapist can control these movements by placing her hands about the head of the humerus with the fingers in the axilla pressing outward against the head of the humerus (Fig. 44).

The patient should be taught to roll from side to side which

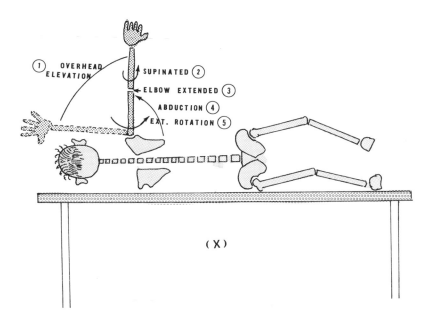

FIGURE 43. In passive exercise, the patient tries to hold the extremity in various positions (1–5).

initiates trunk movements, facilitates nursing care such as bed making, and prevents pressure sores. During rolling the arm must not be permitted to retract, i.e., flex backward. The patient's head must also not be permitted to flex laterally toward the affected side. This requires proper positioning of the patient's head or removal of the pillow. Total body rolling promotes awareness of the body, initiates reflex activity in the extremities, decreases spasticity, and begins the road to self-care.

When the patient begins regaining trunk control, he then is seated at the edge of the bed balancing by use of the sound arm. Gradually, the patient is caused to lean toward the affected side supporting his body weight upon the affected arm. Weight bearing upon the elbow is first begun with arm flexed. Gradually weight bearing upon the wrist and palm with elbow extended and hand turned outward is attempted. When the patient's active cooperation becomes evident, the patient's arm should passively, then actively assist to move in:

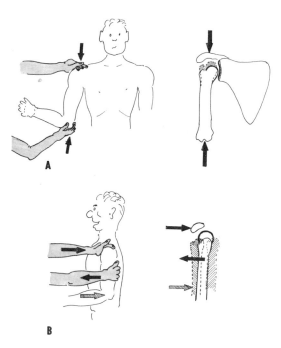

FIGURE 44. Mobilization of the shoulder to regain joint play. *A,* Traction-compression forces against humerus. *B,* Anteroposterior mo-

1. An externally rotated direction
2. Shoulder flexed forward and upward
3. Elbow extended
4. Wrist extended, the fingers extended, and thumb abducted

This arm position should be maintained as much as possible whether patient is supine, side lying, rolling over, or ultimately sitting and standing.

Because the deltoid is considered to belong to the extensor synergy,[4] ultimate contraction of the deltoid is facilitated by ensuring the total extensor pattern of the upper extremity. When the patient attempts to sit, he should be encouraged to support his *weight on the affected side* with the extended arm that is

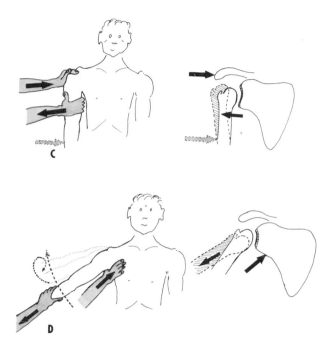

bilization of glenohumeral joint. *C,* Abduction mobilization. *D,* Rotatory mobilization.

simultaneously abducted, externally rotated, with the fingers extended and thumb abducted (Fig. 45).

SUBLUXATION OF THE SHOULDER

One of the perplexing complications of the hemiplegic shoulder is the subluxation of the glenohumeral joint. Subluxation may be noted early in the flail shoulder, may be first noted in early spasticity, or may complicate the chronic severe spastic extremity. It has been related to sensory impairment but has been noted in patients who do not have apparent sensory deficit. It may be painless although it more frequently is painful. The exact causative factors remain problematic.

In 1952, Bierman and Licht[5] considered subluxation of the shoulder as a cause of pain, disability, and ultimate frozen shoul-

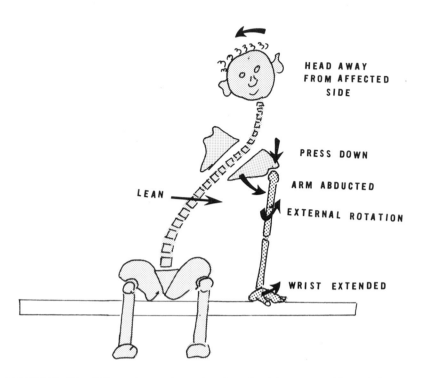

HEAD AWAY
FROM AFFECTED
SIDE

PRESS DOWN

ARM ABDUCTED

LEAN

EXTERNAL ROTATION

WRIST EXTENDED

FIGURE 45. When the patient sits, he should support his weight on the affected side in the manner depicted.

der. This was corroborated by Tobis[6] who felt that the stretched shoulder capsule and cuff muscles were contributing factors. Both advocated a supporting sling.

As was mentioned in Chapter 2, the glenohumeral joint stability is maintained mechanically by:

1. The angle of the glenoid fossa: viz, facing forward, upward and outward, which, therefore, depends on
2. The proper support of the scapula upon the rib cage
3. The mechanical seating of the head of the humerus passively by the supraspinatus fraction of the rotation cuff
4. Possible support from the superior portion of the capsule and
5. Contraction of the deltoid and the cuff muscles when passive support is eliminated by slight abduction of the humerus

Any change in these factors may be instrumental in subluxation.

64

Diagnosis of subluxation is clinical in that the suprahumeral space can be palpated and found to be more elongated than in the opposite normal side. As standardized criteria of subluxation are not yet established, early diagnosis is infrequent and objective evaluation of treatment efficacy is difficult to substantiate. X-ray measurement of subluxation also is comparative. Exact measurement criteria and standards do not exist.

Of the many theories of causation, several merit further evaluation.

1. During the flaccid stage, especially when there is sensory proprioceptive impairment, the cuff muscles (especially the supraspinatus) can be elongated. The "seating" function of the cuff muscles is lost and the head of the humerus can, and does, glide downward as well as laterally.

2. In the early hemiplegic stage the scapula assumes a depressed position. The lowering of the outer aspect of the scapula changes the angulation of the glenoid fossa causing it to be malaligned for the humeral head (Fig. 46).

3. With the usual functional scoliosis that occurs in the hemiplegic, that is, leaning toward the hemiplegic side, the scapula is relatively depressed and rotated. This changes the angulation of the glenoid fossa (Fig. 47).

4. Spasticity of the latissimus dorsi depresses the scapula and places traction as well as internal rotation forces upon the humerus.

5. Paresis of the serratus may contribute to scapular angle change.

6. Spasticity of the scapular muscles, such as the rhomboids and/or levator scapula, can influence subluxation of the glenohumeral joint by depressing and rotating the scapula downward (Fig. 48).

7. Brachial plexus injury complicating the hemiparesis can cause paresis that impairs cuff muscles and scapular muscles with potential subluxation.

65

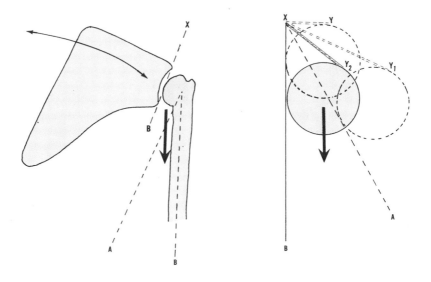

FIGURE 46. Mechanism of glenohumeral subluxation. Left figure depicts change of glenoid angle X–B when scapula is rotated. The humerus becomes abducted (B) and subluxes downward. Right figure shows "seating" of the head of the humerus supported by cuff X–Y$_1$ when glenoid angle is physiologic X–A. When scapula rotates, the angle becomes vertical X–B, and the cuff no longer "seats" the head X–Y$_2$. The humerus subluxes downward.

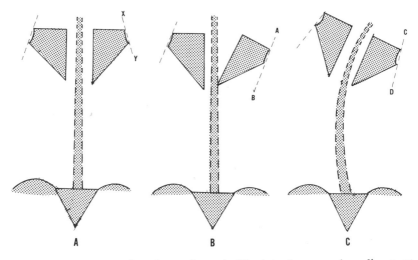

FIGURE 47. Scapular depression. A, Depicts the scapular alignment with a straight spine (X–Y glenoid angle). B, Paresis with downward rotation of the scapula (A–B glenoid angle). C, Relative downward rotation of scapula with functional scoliosis (C–D glenoid angle).

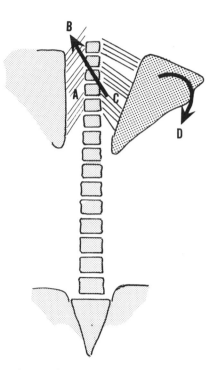

FIGURE 48. Spastic medial scapular muscles. In spasm of the rhomboid muscles that normally rotate the scapula, the glenoid fossa alignment is lowered and the angulation made vertical.

Treatment

Of the various treatments advocated for the subluxed shoulder, support by a sling has had the most proponents and also has the greatest controversy. There are numerous designs, all postulating mechanical advantages (Fig. 49). Hurd and associates[7] concluded that the commonly used hemisling had no appreciable effect on ultimate range of motion, subluxation, pain, or peripheral nerve traction injury. There are many who claim that a sling contributes to subluxation rather than preventing it, encourages flexor synergy by maintaining the arm in flexed position, and inhibits extension. There are claims that a sling impairs the body image both psychologically as well as physiologically and impairs body balance in walking or arising from a seated position. In walking, it supposedly inhibits arm swing in developing a good

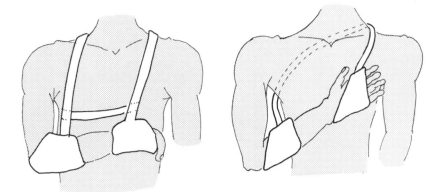

FIGURE 49. Shoulder slings. These slings are designed to support the arm and minimize downward subluxation of the glenohumeral joint. They have not been proven to prevent subluxation and hold the arm in a flex position.

gait pattern. The Rood sling was designed to be dynamic in that by virtue of the elastic support it offers proprioceptive stimulation by forcing the head of the humerus up into the suprahumeral arch (Figs. 50 and 51). Patients whose stroke confines them to a wheelchair may have the arm supported by an overhead sling that purportedly prevents edema and permits active and passive range of motion. The sling also minimizes subluxation of the shoulder as well as preventing painful disabling deformities of the wrist and fingers (Fig. 52).

SUMMARY

In addition to the use of a sling, if that is the decision of the therapist, the scapula must be mobilized to laterally displace its inferior angle. The glenohumeral joint range of motion must be maintained passively and when any muscle tone returns every attempt to regain voluntary motion must be utilized.

With the onset of spasticity, emphasis must be on preventing internal rotation and adduction. The latissimus dorsi must be

68

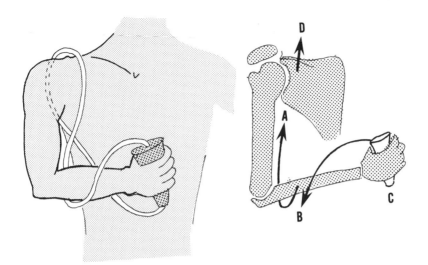

FIGURE 50. Rood sling. The support being elastic tubing gives kinetic support (A) and stimulates extension of the arm. By proper application, the forearm is supinated (B). The hand is held in a cone (C) that spreads the fingers and thumb while radially deviating the wrist. The scapula is elevated and derotated (D).

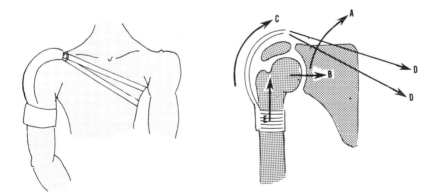

FIGURE 51. Proposed design for prevention of subluxation. A, The glenohumeral joint is elevated to the desired physiologic angulation. B, The head of the humerus is adducted into the "seated" position. C, The humerus is elevated into the suprahumeral fossa. D, The cuff is replaced by the splint. E, The sling attaches to the humerus at the site of deltoid insertion and elevates the humerus into the suprahumeral joint space.

69

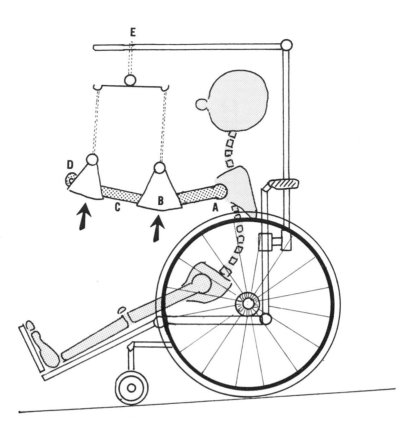

FIGURE 52. Wheel chair arm sling. *A*, Holds shoulder forward, flexed, and adducted. *B*, Supports elbow in an extended position. *C*, *D*, Wrist and fingers held extended. *E*, Permits movement of entire arm.

kept fully elongated. Scoliosis must be minimized by passive and active trunk exercises. Downward and lateral forces upon the glenohumeral joint must be minimized. This is done by using techniques and positions to force the humeral head into the supra-humeral space. Every stimulation technique—tapping, brushing, ice, tonic neck reflexes, and biofeedback—must be attempted and utilized until some voluntary or reflex activity hopefully returns.

REFERENCES

1. Magnus, R., and de Kleijn, A.: Die Abhangigkeib Des Tonus der Ex-tremitatenmuskeln von der Kipfstellung. Arch. Physiol. (Pfluegers) 154:455–548, 1912.

2. McCoach, G. P., Deering, I. D., and Ling, T. H.: Location of receptors for tonic neck reflexes. J. Neurophysiol. 14:191–195, 1951.
3. Johnstone, M.: The Stroke Patient: Principles of Rehabilitation. Churchill Livingstone, London, 1976.
4. Bobath, B.: Adult Hemiplegia: Evaluation and Treatment, ed. 2. Heineman Medical Books, London, 1978.
5. Bierman, W., and Licht, S. (eds.): Physical Medicine in General Practice, ed. 3. Hoeber, New York, 1952, p. 601.
6. Tobis, J. S.: Post-hemiplegic shoulder pain. N.Y.J. Med. 57:1377–1380, 1957.
7. Hurd, M. M., Farrell, K. H., and Waylonis, G. W.: Shoulder sling for hemiplegia: friend or foe? Arch. Phys. Med. Rehabil. 55:519, Nov. 1974.

CHAPTER 4

Spastic Stage

The flaccid stage usually evolves into the spastic stage. Spasticity has an insidious onset with the flexors of the arm and the extensors of the leg being predominantly involved. In the upper extremity the shoulder girdle depressors and the fixators of the scapulae are involved early. Almost simultaneously the adductors (pectoralis major, latissimus dorsi, teres minor and major, and the subscapularis and infraspinatus) become spastic. Distally the upper extremity assumes the usual pattern of spasticity with flexion and pronation of the elbow and flexion of the wrist and fingers.[1]

Passive resistance of a specific proximal movement depends to a large degree on position of the distal portion of the arm. An example is arm elevation which is much more limited by spasticity with the arm externally rotated and the elbow extended than when the movement is attempted with arm internally rotated and the elbow flexed.

With severe neurologic involvement, movement of the arm is greatly affected by the position of the head and neck. The arm may extend at the elbow with the head turned toward that side, and flex at the elbow when the head is turned away from the involved side. The arms may assume the extended position when the head and neck are extended and assume the flexor pattern when flexed. These are the classic tonic neck reflexes. After the

73

flail stage of hemiplegia, severely involved patients may remain at the synergistic stage in which, either by reflex or attempted voluntary action, gross synergistic movements result. Total inability to perform individual movements or any individual components of the synergy ultimately develops.

As most patients sooner or later evolve from the flaccid stage into the spastic stage, there is gradual entry into the patterns of synergy. These patterns are stereotyped and can be initiated as reflexes as well as be initiated by voluntary actions. Of the two synergies, there are few variations in respect to the shoulder or elbow other than the relative strength of either of the pattern components. The hand, wrist, and fingers vary in the synergistic patterns and cannot be considered as consistent patterns.

With further loss of cortical control, the emergence of synergies becomes apparent.[2] Flexor synergy predominantly prevails in the upper extremity. Flexor synergies of the upper extremity consist of:

1. Elbow flexed at an acute angle
2. Abduction of the shoulder to 90°
3. External rotation of the shoulder
4. Supination of the forearm
5. Retraction or elevation of the scapula

The synergies basically are neurophysiologic patterns of the middle motor centers.[2] This is compared to the extensor synergy of the upper extremity in which there is:

1. Protraction of the scapula
2. Forward flexion of the arm toward the front of the body
3. Internal rotation of the arm
4. Extension of the elbow
5. Pronation of the forearm

With the emergence of synergies in the stroke sequence, any specific component of the flexor synergy may be elicited in the extensor synergy and vice versa.

Upon entering the spastic stage, the hemiplegic patient usually

74

exhibits elbow flexion first. This aspect of the flexor synergy is the strongest. The shoulder phase of the synergy is weaker and may never appear unless the patient progresses into a more reflex status or regains more voluntary control.

When the hemiplegic patient attempts to abduct the upper extremity, only certain movements are possible. The shoulder girdle elevates but there is very little abduction of the glenohumeral joint. The scapular adductors may prevent the scapula from moving forward in an attempt to elevate and forward flex the arm. This presents a therapeutic problem in that they must be passively stretched. The stroke patient may never regain abduction or external rotation of the arm. The arm assumes posterior flexion instead.

In extensor synergy of the upper extremity, the strongest component is the pectoralis major. In the transition between the flaccid and spastic phases, spasticity frequently is first noted in the pectoralis major. Spasticity of the forearm pronators occurs next in sequence, but usually appears later. This posture of an adducted, internally rotated arm with flexed elbow and pronated forearm is considered to be the "typical arm pattern" of the hemiplegic.

Movement of the arm may be affected by the position of the head and neck, but these tonic neck and labyrinthine reflexes, which were originally noted in decerebrate animals, are only of great value in very severely involved humans. They should, however, be tested in patients and utilized whenever they have application.

Trunk movements have also been found to influence extremity movements. Rotation of the upper trunk upon the lower trunk facilitates or inhibits reflex patterns as well as voluntary patterns and should also be clinically evaluated. It has been shown that rotation of the upper trunk facilitates flexion of the side toward which there is rotation and extension of the side away from which there is rotation.[3]

It appears from review of the literature that associated patterns are reinforced with simultaneous head-neck positions. Thus, as a patient is asked to contract a certain muscle group against resistance, the head and neck position should be varied toward or away from the involved side. The trunk rotation should also be varied and the patient tested in a lying and/or sitting position.[4,5]

Hemiplegic patients frequently exhibit associated reactions in which active volunteer movement of the uninvolved side causes movement of the involved side and resistance of the active movement of the ipsilateral extremity is apt to elicit associated reactions. These associated reactions can occur when the involved side is flaccid or has sensory impairment. There are no consistent patterns to be elicited, but trial of various components of the normal extremity movement patterns must be attempted in the hope of initiating movements. Albeit, these movements may be reflex but will initiate movement in the normally flaccid extremity. It has been claimed by many clinical investigators, however, that reflex patterns so elicited rarely come under voluntary control. With today's interest in biofeedback, new treatment techniques may emerge that will have functional significance.

There may be severe, mild, or subtle sensory impairment that may cause the patient's inability to use the upper extremity. This sensory impairment must often be specifically tested in a manner that may not affect the involved side. The patient may fail to recognize the affected side. When he or she is asked to draw a human body, the involved side is frequently not drawn (Fig. 53).

The patient may have astereognosis in which he or she fails to recognize familiar objects such as coins, keys, pins, pens, and so forth by touch or feel. Agnosia may be present in which the patient recognizes the shape, size, texture, and so on of an object but cannot give its name or its use. There may be a unilateral visual deficit, decreased level of awareness, or poor cooperation. All of these impairments inhibit function and influence the prognosis of recovery.[6]

Even a diminished regain of function or dexterity and pain-free movement of the upper extremity can facilitate transfer activities such as rolling over in bed and gross self-care function.

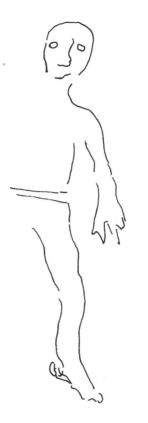

FIGURE 53. Denial demonstrated by patient. When a patient is asked to draw his body or a person, he is aware of only one half of his body, denying the existence of the other half. This is such a drawing from a patient.

As voluntary control returns, portions of the synergies are isolated and stressed in treatment with the purpose of separating them from other components of the synergy. As an example, arm elevation is attempted without simultaneous elbow flexion and, once isolated, is stressed in treatment.

All movements normally are responses to the sensory stimulus which acts through exteroceptors, vision, touch, and hearing. The proprioceptors send their sensory messages from the muscles, tendons, joints, and skin. In many hemiplegic patients, there may be a varying degree of sensory deficit which impairs voluntary movement and hinders therapeutic attempts.

The Bobaths[10] feel that the hemiplegic problem is not a lack of muscle power but the patient's inability to control isolated or voluntary components of the pattern. The hemiplegic patterns are few and stereotyped and are in essence gross synergies. The Bobaths' techniques are "to change abnormal patterns of movement" and they claim that therapy should avoid heavy resistance exercises, such as those claimed to be effective by Walters[7] or Knott[8] in the PNF technique. The Bobaths also are opposed to the use of Brunnstrom's associated reactions[9] which they feel should be avoided in the upper motor neuron lesions. They claim that these techniques reinforce synergies and thus increase spasticity. They feel that coordination cannot be utilized so long as massive reflex tonic patterns of the synergy remain and the basic tonic reflexes still predominate.[10]

The Bobaths' concepts of muscular weakness are as follows:

1. The weakness is due to being relatively overcome by overwhelming spastic antagonistic muscles.
2. A muscle may be weak only as a prime mover but "strong" whenever an abnormal mass movement pattern occurs.
3. Weakness may be caused by sensory deficit.
4. Soft tissue periarticular contraction can enhance or simulate weakness.

The Bobaths feel that the problem of spasticity and the synergies must be prevented or controlled before voluntary motor activity can be achieved.[10] They claim this may be achieved by "special handling" of the patient and this handling can be done by controlling certain aspects of the pattern which they call the "key points" of control. These key points are the proximal neck, spine, shoulder, and pelvic aspects of the pattern. An important key point in the upper extremity is rotation of the shoulder girdle toward the spine. Total rotation of the shoulder girdle in relationship to the trunk and pelvis is thus an important aspect of the Bobath's theory, as is neck rotation in relationship to the pelvis and/or the shoulder-arm patterns.

78

In the hemiplegic patient, there is no reciprocal relaxation of the antagonist by agonist contraction, instead there is cocontraction. Muscle reeducation with biofeedback is currently used to learn to relax the spastic antagonist and thus release the prime movers. It is conceivable that eventually biofeedback can be applied to muscular reeducation of the agonist with simultaneous inhibition of antagonist muscle activity. Relaxation of the antagonist currently can be done by nerve block techniques, either by local anesthetic or by injecting dilute phenol in the motor points of the spastic antagonist muscles.

The muscles that are initially affected in spasticity are the depressors and fixators of the scapula. These muscles prevent active movement of the arm in the desired direction. The depressors are more powerful than the elevators, thus the upper extremity assumes scapular depression and adduction, internal rotation of arm flexion of the elbow, and pronation of the forearm. The pronator group of the forearm muscles includes, in this flexor synergy, the flexor carpi radialis and wrist flexors. The remainder of the flexor synergy is wrist flexion and finger flexion. These distal components of the pattern must be controlled in retraining the proximal portion of the pattern. In passively attempting to abduct the arm and elevate the arm above horizontal, there is resistance of adduction at the glenohumeral joint, internal rotation of the arm, and rotation of the scapula.

When the patient is beginning sitting balance exercises, the arm must always be held in the proper position and pressure exerted upward into the glenohumeral joint. This acts as a proprioceptive stimulus as the patient is pushed off balance[10,11] or is made to be off balance. Traction upon the affected arm may promote some motor response, but approximation with pressure *upward* stimulates postural reflexes.

TECHNIQUES OF MUSCLE REEDUCATION

Without stressing one concept of treatment over another but utilizing the basic concepts of all, a "technique" can be summarized. If relaxation is required, focus patient's attention on the agonist or antagonist by the following techniques:

1. Visualization of muscle group and movement using a mirror. May be demonstrated to the patient by the therapist.

2. Passive movement of the shoulder in abduction, forward flexion, and external rotation combined with visualization (mirror) or by verbal commands of the therapist.

3. Similar movement of the other (normal) shoulder done separately for instruction or simultaneously with passive movement of the involved shoulder.

4. Encouraging patient to "feel where arm is," "feel the muscles that move the shoulder," or "feel the movement." Pain here, if present, must be eliminated or minimized.

5. Place arm in an antigravity position then have patient "hold" in that acquired position.

6. To decrease the depression and retraction of the shoulder girdle, the affected hand is placed on the opposite shoulder and the elbow is elevated to the horizontal position.

7. Upward retraction (forcing shoulder up into the subacromial area). Place the entire arm in a fully extended, slightly externally rotated position *with wrist and fingers extended*. In a spastic state, traction may initiate the desired movement. Both should be tried (traction and retraction) to determine which is the most effective. Using a supporting sling prevents traction and, in fact, encourages dependency. Adduction and internal rotation, such as in the Rood sling, has some approximation stimulation.

8. Apply simultaneous skin sensation over the muscle belly. Light rubbing, brushing, ice application, tapping, muscle kneading, or brisk rubbing of the agonist stimulate contraction. This sensor stimulation should be done with simultaneous verbal and visual stimulation.[12]

9. Shoulder girdle elevation and depression is performed actively if the patient is able to initiate this movement. If the patient is unable, the extended arm is passively used to ele-

vate the girdle with simultaneous percussion or cutaneous stimulation of the upper trapezius.[14]

Prone exercises plus kneeling encourage approximation so that when sitting, lying prone, crawling, or kneeling is done with the affected arm bearing weight, the desired pattern is encouraged (Figs. 54 and 55).

10. Relaxation of spastic antagonist must be accomplished by:

    a. Increasing range passively with slow gentle stretching to avoid stimulation of the stretch reflex. This is done simultaneously with ice application to the spastic muscle.

    b. Contraction of the spastic antagonist followed immediately by relaxation (verbal) then immediate gentle passive stretching of that antagonist.

    c. Alternate contraction of agonist, then antagonist, then agonist—done verbally, with or without traction—with

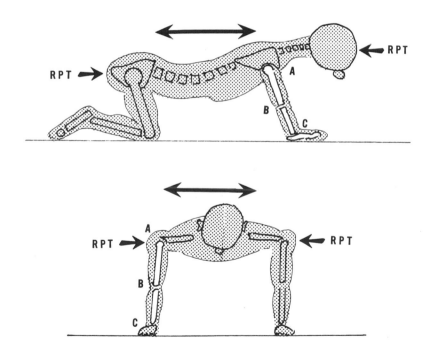

FIGURE 54. Patient crawling with weight-bearing on affected arm. RPT-indicates resisted pressure from therapist.

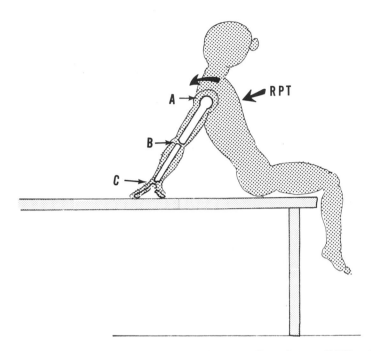

FIGURE 55. Patient sitting and leaning on affected arm. RPT-patient resists pressure from therapist.

total arm involvement (wrist, fingers, and elbows). This is often best done in PNF patterns (overhead elevation, abduction, internal rotation, that is, palm facing backward and thumb out with elbow, wrist, fingers extended, then downward across chest with internal rotation and wrist and fingers flexed). This "rhythmic stabilization" must be done slowly to insure the patient's cooperation (Figs. 56 and 57).

11. Vigorous stretching of the spastic muscles stretches the connective tissues of the muscles and the tendon organs which supposedly decreases muscle spindle activity.[12] Vigorous stretching also stretches the tendon organs which inhibits alpha and gamma neurons which reflexly relaxes the muscle.[13]

12. Electrical stimulation of the antagonist relaxes these muscles in some cases.

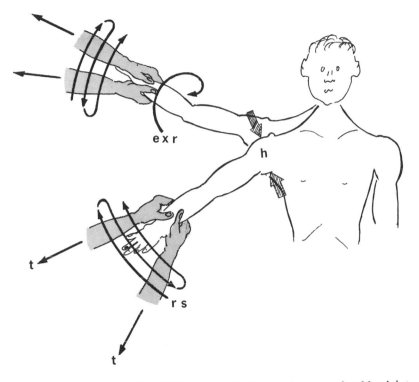

FIGURE 56. Rhythmic stabilization technique to increase shoulder joint range of motion. As the therapist elevates, abducts, and externally rotates (exr) the arm with some traction (t), the patient resists to prevent motion. The exact opposite motion of the arm is then attempted by the therapist and resisted by the patient. As shown in Figure 57, the same amount of force and resistance must be exerted by the therapist as by the patient. Minimal joint motion occurs (h) and most muscular contraction is isometric.

13. Bilateral training in which the normal arm is exercised simultaneously with the paretic arm. This has been advocated but not with specific emphasis on the shoulder. In the forearm exercises of pronation and supination, the normal side becomes erratic when the paretic side is exercised, implying that the damaged cortex may impair the function of the uninvolved side. After a stroke, the nonparetic side has been postulated to compete with the paretic side during bilateral movements. Further studies are warranted before bilateral symmetrical patterns are used in treatment.

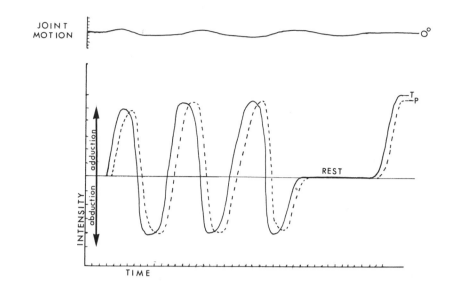

FIGURE 57. Alternating cycle of rhythmic stabilization. The force exerted by the therapist (T) must be equally resisted by the patient (P). Contraction is isometric. After a brief series of alternating contractions, the shoulder is relaxed and a new position is gained passively by the therapist, hence gaining an increased range of motion.

14. "Tight" muscle fibers that develop in spastic muscles create "trigger areas" that maintain the spasticity and the contracture. These trigger areas can be dispelled by deep finger pressure, ultrasound, or local electrical pressure.

15. Use of modalities, especially ice application, will often decrease spasticity and allow greater active and passive range of motion.[15]

The variables in these techniques are sensory loss, conceptual impairment, flaccidity or spasticity, and numerous other impairments. Furthermore, the position of the patient must be varied to utilize neck positions, trunk positions, and prone or supine positions as these may enhance or inhibit the exercises. Numerous treatment sessions are needed for complete evaluation of the hemiplegic patient.

Biofeedback is still in its early research phase and has potential merit. In any physical therapy regimen, feedback consists of verbal, visual, and sensory responses. Electromyographic feed-

84

back also employs these responses. A recent preliminary evaluation of EMG feedback efficacy versus "standard" physical therapy implies that EMG retrains only a limited number of motor elements rather than encouraging function.[16] Patients with perceptual deficits will not benefit as much as nonimpaired patients. All patients considered to be candidates for rehabilitation or neuromuscular rehabilitation must be evaluated for perceptual deficits.[17,18] Brain defined those with perceptual deficits as "people who were guessing the meaning of a language for which they did not know the alphabet."[19]

Functional evaluation and classification, including perception, must be systematically performed and documented,[20,21] otherwise no technique of reeducation will be wholly effective. Before any battery of tests is given, it is mandatory that the patient be evaluated to see if the conclusion drawn will be valid and to determine his perceptual abilities. The following must be investigated:

1. Mental status.
    a. Orientation as to time, place, and person.
    b. Memory, specifically immediate recall or short-term memory.
    c. Attention span: thus the ability to concentrate on the test.
    d. Effect of the patient's behavior toward the test.
2. Apraxia which may be confused with perceptual defect.
3. Premorbid medical status such as hearing, speech, and vision.

"Predictive factors" to determine the outcome of stroke, either from natural recovery or from treatment, are not yet well documented. Correlation of functional impairment with anatomic site of pathology is also not clarified, so a precise neurologic localization of pathology does not prognosticate degree nor rapidity of recovery.[23,24]

There is no validity to the postulate that left hemiparesis presents greater disability than right hemiparesis or vice versa. Excessive spasticity is an accepted poor prognostic factor as is the presence of nystagmus, impaired visuospacial perception, constructional dyspraxia, spacial agnosia, or pseudobulbar palsy. Sensory impairment is a recognized negative prognostic factor.[25]

Peripheral sensation must be intact before cortical sensory interpretation can be validated. If the patient has impaired peripheral sensation, he cannot be expected to perceive what he is feeling. Without peripheral sensation, testing for stereognosis (identifying objects) or two point discrimination (when one point cannot be felt) cannot be accurately evaluated. Even body image, such as identifying different parts of the body, cannot be tested when peripheral sensation is impaired.

It becomes apparent that a "standard" method or technique of muscle reeducation cannot be applied to all patients. Every technique merits consideration and evaluation until the most effective technique for that patient is found.

REFERENCES

1. Beevor, C. E.: The Croonian Lectures. Adlard and Son, London, 1904.
2. Jackson, J. H.: On some implications of dissolution of the nervous system. Med. Press Circular, 2:411, 1882.
3. Tokizane, T., Muras, M., Ogata, T., et al.: Electromyographic studies in tonic neck, lumbar and labyrinthic reflexes in normal persons. Jap. J. Physiol. 2:130, 1951.
4. Simons, A.: Kapfhaltang and Muskeltonus, Felinische Biobachtanges. Z. Neurol. 80:499, 1923.
5. Brunnstrom, S.: Movement Therapy in Hemiplegia: A Neurophysiological Approach. Harper and Row, New York, 1970.
6. Caldwell, C. B., Wilson, D. J., and Braun, R. M.: Evaluation and treatment in the hemiplegic stroke patient. Clin. Orthop. 63:69, March–April, 1969.
7. Walters, C. E.: Interaction of the body and its segments. Am. J. Phys. Med. 46:1, 1967.
8. Knott, M.: Introduction to and philosophy of neuromuscular facilitation. Physiotherapy, 53:1, 1967.
9. Brunnstrom, S.: Associated reactions of the upper extremity in adult patients with hemiplegia. Phys. Ther. Rev. 35:4, 1956.
10. Bobath, B.: Adult Hemiplegia: Evaluation and Treatment. William Heinemann Medical Book Ltd., London, 1970.
11. Rood, M.: Neurophysiological Reactions as a Basis for Physical Therapy. Phys. Ther. Rev. 34:444, 1954.
12. Kottke, F. J.: Neurophysiological Therapy for Stroke and Its Rehabilitation, Licht, S. (ed.). Waverly Press, Baltimore, 1975.
13. Bobath, K., and Bobath, B.: Spastic paralysis treatment by the use of reflex inhibition. Brit. J. Phys. Med. 13:121, 1950.
14. Keelan, V.: Letters to editor. Phys. Ther. 52:1209, Nov. 1972.

15. Showman, J., and Wedlich, L.: The use of cold instead of heat for the relief of muscle spasm. Med. J. Aust. 2:15, 1963.
16. Mroczek, N., Halpern, D., and McHugh, R.: Electromyographic feedback and physical therapy for neuromuscular retraining in hemiplegia. Arch. Phys. Med. Rehab. 59:258, June 1978.
17. Jimenez, J., Keltz, E., Stein, M. C., et al.: Evaluation of stroke disability. Can. Med. Assoc. J. 114:615, April 1976.
18. Strub, R. L., and Black, F. W.: The Mental Status Examination in Neurology. F. A. Davis Co., Philadelphia, 1977.
19. Brain, W. R.: Mind Perception and Science. Blackwell, Oxford, England, 1951.
20. Jiminez, J., Caiarcossi, A., Keltz, E. et al.: Prerequisites for perceptual evaluation on brain damage. Can. Med. Assoc. J. 115 (12):165, Dec. 1976.
21. Anderson, T. P., Boubestrom, N., Greenberg, F. R., et al.: Predictive factors in stroke rehabilitation. Arch. Phys. Med. Rehab. 55:545, 1974.
22. Adams, G. F., and Hurwitz, L. J.: Mental barriers to recovery from strokes. Lancet 2:533, 1963.
23. Gordon, E. E., Drenth, V., Jarvis, L., et al.: Neurophysiologic syndromes in stroke as predictors of outcome. Arch. Phys. Med. Rehabil. 59:399, Sept. 1978.
24. Cain, L. S.: Determining factors that affect rehabilitation. Am. J. Geriatr. Soc. 17:595, 1969.
25. Ayres, A. J.: Perception of space of adult hemiplegic patients. Arch. Phys. Med. Rehabil. 43:552, 1962.

CHAPTER 5

The Painful Shoulder

The shoulder of the hemiplegic patient may be painful and present an additional problem in treatment of stroke. The pain may be directly related to the neurologic impairment of the hemiplegia or may be the result of the many causes of shoulder pain in the nonhemiplegic.[1] The pain resulting from attrition, inflammation, or previous trauma may have been latent but activated by the hemiplegia. Numerous names have been applied to the painful shoulder:[2] supraspinatus tendonitis, rotator cuff tendonitis, subacromial bursitis, subdeltoid bursitis, painful arc syndrome, calcific tendonitis, calcific bicipital tendonitis, periarthritis, adhesive capsulitis, frozen shoulder, adhesive bursitis, periarticular adhesives, and check rein shoulder.

Codman[3] initially attributed the painful limited shoulder to a localized supraspinatus tendonitis which led to inflammation of the other components of the cuff, to the adjacent subacromial bursa with extension into the joint capsule, and ultimately to inflammation of all the intra-articular tissues leading to a frozen shoulder. Many of these stages are still considered relevant in the sequence of the painful shoulder, but hemiplegia adds a new or different dimension to the painful shoulder and to the limitation leading to the frozen shoulder. Pain leading to immobilization ultimately leads to disuse atrophy, contracture, osteoporosis, and varying degrees of disability[3,4] (Fig. 58).

89

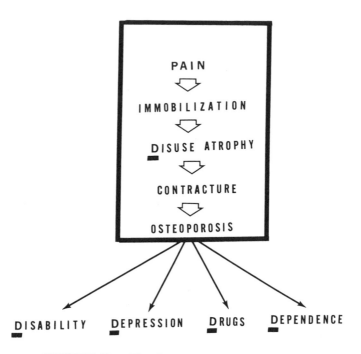

FIGURE 58.   The five *D*s resulting from pain.

The etiology of tendonitis has been attributed to ischemia by some investigators and to hyperemia by others.[5] The circulation of the cuff muscles and tendons, especially the supraspinatus muscle, has been reasonably ascertained to be either ischemic or hyperemic, depending upon external forces (Fig. 59). In the "critical" zone of the supraspinatus tendon, there is a large vascular anastomosis that brings abundant circulation when the tendon is relaxed and not compressed. Tension upon the tendon when the arm is dependent or is tensed by the contracting muscles during active motion causes local ischemia. Compression between the tuberosities and the acromion can also cause ischemia. After the age of 50, the supraspinatus tendon undergoes thinning, fraying, fissuring, and fibrillation within the critical zone. This undoubtedly is a process of attrition enhanced by intermittent ischemia and hyperemia.

Calcium deposits attributed to the inevitable sequelae of degeneration are not usually present. Mucopolysaccharides in nor-

90

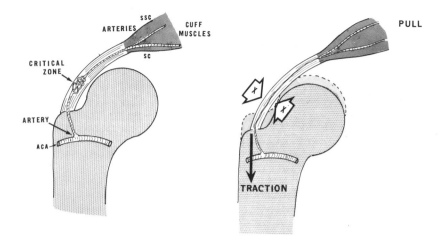

FIGURE 59. Circulation to the critical zone of the supraspinatus tendon. When the arm is relaxed and supported, the critical zone has abundant circulation. Traction from the dependent arm or from contraction of the cuff muscles compresses the tendon (at site X–X), and the zone becomes ischemic. ACA = anterior circumflex artery; SSC = suprascapular artery; SC = subscapular artery.

mal cartilage inhibit calcification. However, any pathology that depletes mucopolysaccharides allows calcification to occur. Calcific tendonitis is reported in 8 percent of nonsymptomatic population over the age of 30.[5] It is estimated that 35 percent of all calcific deposits cause some symptoms. Codman[3] concluded that any calcific deposit larger than 1.5 cm. in diameter would be symptomatic, thus 35 percent of all calcific deposits have been concluded to be of that size. It is of interest that those calcific deposits considered to be an end stage of degeneration are rarely associated with complete rotator cuff tears.[7] For apparently mechanical reasons, subscapularis tendon calcium deposits are usually asymptomatic.

The painful shoulder requires a careful examination to ascertain the site and tissue cause of pain. This is true in the non-hemiplegic patient as well as in the hemiplegic. Steindler[8] specified sites of tissue pain as illustrated in Figure 60. The site of pain and the tissue responsible can be specified by palpation, muscle examination, and observation of the scapulohumeral movement

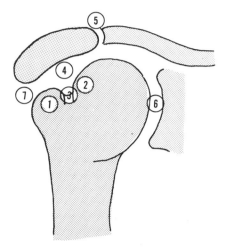

FIGURE 60. Sites of tissue pain. *1*, Greater tuberosity: attachment of supraspinatus tendon. *2*, Lesser tuberosity. *3*, Bicipital groove: tendon of long head of biceps. *4*, Subacromial bursa. *5*, Acromioclavicular joint. *6*, Glenohumeral joint and capsule. *7*, Subdeltoid bursa. (Modified from Steindler.[8])

on active motion. The history stated by the patient usually localizes the site of pain and the specific motion causing it. This is not always possible in the hemiplegic as there may be lack of verbal communication and there may be markedly impaired voluntary shoulder function from either flaccidity or spasticity.

Much of the examination of a hemiplegic patient is done passively or with limited active participation. In spite of these restrictions, a very meaningful examination is possible. Radiologic examinations are of limited value as a rule unless fracture or dislocation are suspected, but their value merits consideration.

RADIOLOGIC EXAMINATION

There are changes noted on conventional x-rays that are significant in determining the cause of shoulder pain or dysfunction.[9]

1. Cystic changes in the tuberosities are the earliest detectable x-ray changes revealing attritional changes. These were described by Codman[3] as cysts or "caverns containing vascular tissue."

92

These cysts are probably the result of bony changes resulting from repeated traction from the supraspinatus tendon (Fig. 61, top).

2. Erosion of the tuberosities of the humerus gradually results from the wear and tear from rubbing under surface of the coracoacromial arch. The tuberosities become walled over the cysts and then erode causing a "volcano" appearance (Fig. 61, bottom).

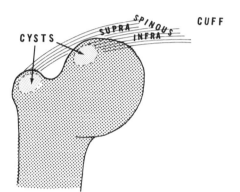

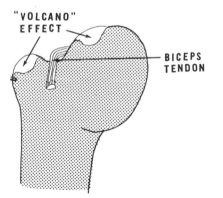

FIGURE 61. Roentgenographic changes in shoulder dysfunction: cysts in the tuberosities of the humerus. These are early x-ray evidence of attrition. With wear and tear, the tuberosities become eroded causing a volcano appearance. The bicipital groove becomes shallow.

93

With erosion, the bicipital groove, formed by the greater and lesser tuberosities, becomes more shallow permitting subluxation of the biceps tendon. This subluxation can cause pain: the so-called bicipital tendinitis syndrome variant.

3. As the tuberosities erode they become replaced by eburnated bone. This is also termed osteophytosis and gradually erodes into the overhanging acromion. Hypertrophy and spur formation from bony overgrowth decrease joint space, decrease joint range of motion, and cause increasing pain (Fig. 62). With gradual disappearance of the tuberosities and increasing shallow-

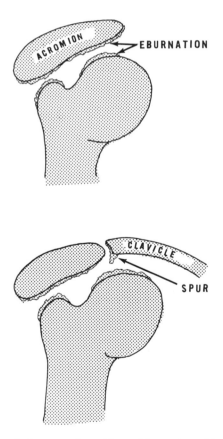

FIGURE 62. Stages of degeneration. Top, The tuberosities disappear and are replaced by eburnated bone. Bottom, In addition to hypertrophic change of the humeral head and the acromion, there are changes in the acromioclavicular joint including spur formation.

ness of the bicipital groove, attrition of the biceps tendon occurs with potential disruption and pain.

ACROMIOCLAVICULAR LESION

Pain can occur from degeneration of the acromioclavicular joint. These symptoms can occur long before or even without x-ray changes of the joint. Pain is noted at the acromioclavicular joint. Tenderness can be elicited over the joint, crepitation can be felt upon movement of the joint, and the movement (elevation and depression of the shoulder girdle "shrugging") without simultaneous glenohumeral movement all specify the site of pain to be at that specific joint. Injection of an anesthetic agent into the joint which relieves the pain is both diagnostic and therapeutic. The acromioclavicular joint is abused to a large degree in hemiplegia because of the limited glenohumeral movement that causes a "shrugging" instead of abduction or forward flexion on attempted arm movement.

BICIPITAL TENDINITIS

This is a frequent cause of shoulder pain that is overlooked when a diagnosis of painful shoulder is evaluated. The long head of the biceps originates at the supraglenoid tubercle on the superior rim of the glenoid fossa. It then proceeds laterally to make a sharp angulation at the bicipital groove of the humerus. The groove is formed by the greater and lesser tuberosities of the head of the humerus. It proceeds between the subscapularis and the supraspinatus tendon in a synovial sheath which is essentially an extension of the shoulder joint capsule. The biceps sheath extends down the bicipital sulcus approximately 5 cm. (2 inches). The biceps tendon does not move in the bicipital groove but rather the bicipital groove moves along the tendon as the arm is moved.

The greatest excursion of the biceps tendon occurs when the arm moves from the internally rotated forward flexed position, is elevated and abducted, then lowered, externally rotated, and posteriorly flexed. This motion pattern is generally the direction of treatment movements performed and encouraged in the hemiplegic patient. Pain can result.

Lippman[9] considered adhesive capsulitis to be rare, but bicipital tenosynovitis to be common. The postulated sequence was mild tenosynovitis of the long head of the biceps, then aggravation of the tenosynovitis, progressing to adhesions. This sequence also postulated that when the adhesions became firm, pain would subside but motion would also become very limited. Motion returns when there is subsidence of the inflammation or there is disintegration of the intraarticular portion of the tendon.

Lesions of the biceps tendon are considered when the following characteristics are noted:

1. There is chronic pain at the anterolateral aspect of the shoulder.
2. Pain is initiated by moving the arm overhead and in an abducted externally rotated direction.
3. Marked to exquisite tenderness exists over the bicipital groove.
4. Pain may be reproduced (localized in the groove) by resisting forward flexion of the shoulder with the elbow extended and the forearm supinated.
5. Feeling and hearing a "click" as the tendon dislocates or moves in and out of the groove.
6. Pain may be reproduced by resisting elbow flexion and supination of the forearm.

CORACOIDITIS

Pain occurring at the coracoid process remains controversial except when there has been direct trauma to the coracoid or discernible traction injury to the tissue attaching to the coracoid. Injury usually has occurred when the arm has been adducted, elevated slightly posteriorly, and externally rotated causing tension in the coracobrachialis and the short head of the biceps.

This syndrome is considered to exist when the pain is localized at the coracoid process (by the patient), frequently occurs at night, is aggravated by abducting, elevating, and externally rotating the arm on resisting the opposite movement, and is elicited over the coracoid process. In the hemiplegic shoulder, this movement (abduction, elevation, and external rotation) is usually markedly restricted. This may be due to spasticity of the involved muscles which causes the arm to be adducted, retracted, and internally rotated, with the elbow flexed and pronated. Although the subscapularis muscle, the prime internal rotator of the arm and an adductor, has been incriminated,[10-12] the coracohumeral ligament undoubtedly retracts within a short while from the persistence of this hemiplegic posture adhesive capsulitis.

Originally the "frozen shoulder" was considered to be caused by adhesive capsulitis with involvement of the biceps tendon.[13] More recent studies do not confirm this assumption but rather consider adhesions of the capsule to be a consequence rather than the cause of the restriction and resultant pain. The frozen shoulder now is considered to be a reflex sympathetic dystrophy which occurs as a result of prolonged immobilization. This immobilization, with pain on active or passive movements, causes autonomic circulatory impairment, muscular and periarticular contracture, and ultimately fibrosis and osteoporosis.

Neviaser[13] performed biopsies of the capsule through arthrotomies and found only 22 percent of patients studied to have subsynovial fibrosis and focal degeneration of collagen that could be construed as capsulitis. The major finding was thickening and contracture of the capsule. Normally the shoulder capsule has a volume of 35 cc. but in adhesive capsulitis the volume decreases to 0.5 to 3.0 cc. and loss of the axillary pouch is noted on arthrography (Fig. 63).

Clinically the frozen shoulder is markedly limited both actively and passively in all ranges of motion. Initially there may be pain, but ultimately pain subsides, restriction of motion increases, and all the shoulder muscles undergo atrophy.

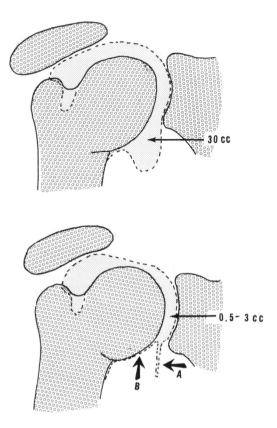

FIGURE 63. Adhesive capsulitis. The normal capsule permits injection of at least 30 cc. of air. In adhesive capsulitis, the capsule adheres to itself (A) and to the humeral head (B). This decreases capacity to 0.5–3 cc. and markedly limits range of motion.

BRACHIAL PLEXIS TRACTION

Traction injury to the brachial plexus is a cause of shoulder pain and dysfunction frequently overlooked. Traction may be the result of a self-incurred injury when the patient moves or is moved while the shoulder and arm are still flaccid. This possibility has been acclaimed as a reason for applying a sling to the flail arm. Clinically, traction injury is suspected when signs and symptoms of peripheral nerve involvement are superimposed upon the hemiplegic paresis.[14] These are manifested by:

98

1. Atypical return of function distally before proximal functional return which is more typical of the hemiparetic sequence.
2. Segmental muscle atrophy consistent with peripheral nerve lesions.
3. Fingers becoming contracted in extension rather than the hemiplegic flexion pattern.
4. Delayed onset of spasticity in the involved muscles.
5. Electromyographic abnormalities indicating lower motor neuron involvement.

DIAGNOSIS

Diagnosis of shoulder pain, either in the hemiplegic or non-hemiplegic patient, is a clinical diagnosis based on:

1. Locating the anatomic site of tissue causing the pain by *palpation*. This requires full knowledge of functional anatomy.
2. Analyzing the active *movement* that reproduces the pain or is prevented by the pain. Here also the muscles, tendons, ligaments, and capsular tissues that are involved and thus cause the pain can be clearly differentiated.
3. *Passive movement* that distinguishes the soft tissue involved.
4. Laboratory confirmation by x-ray, arthrography, or electromyography. Usually a careful clinical examination is diagnostic without need for laboratory confirmation.
5. Local anesthetic infiltration into
   a. suspected soft tissue
   b. nerve supply to tissue
   c. tender trigger area
   confirms the site and tissue causing pain and may be the indication for subsequent treatment.

TREATMENT

The treatment obviously is directly related to relieving the pain emitted from the involved tissues. This may be by oral medica-

99

tion or injected systemic medication. The vast majority of current drugs are antiphlogistic drugs, such as indomethacin, Butazolidin, ibuprofen, or salicylates. The steroids are still valuable, either via the oral or intramuscular route.

Modalities are valuable adjuncts to any treatment regimen. Ice has beneficial effects in relieving the spasms which may cause pain and joint limitation. Ice, preceding pressure or active stretching to increase range of motion, can decrease pain and make the stretching easier. Heat applied locally modifies collagen and fibrous tissue and this facilitates increased range of motion. Ultrasound penetrates more deeply and decreases articular pain. It also slows conduction time of the nerves and theoretically decreases pain transmission.

Exercises, either active or passive, when indicated, are beneficial. In the painful flail extremity, passive ranging is of no value. In the flaccid extremity, the attempt is to restore motor function to regain joint stability and active joint motion. Tapping the muscle or skin stimulation by brushing or stroking over the involved area may indicate motion or muscular contraction that appeared to be impossible. Passively move the arm, then have the patient attempt to "hold" the extremity at the acquired level while stimulating the muscle(s) that would normally move or hold the extremity. Stimulation here consists of tapping, massaging, brushing, or even electrically stimulating the muscle group or groups.

The flail shoulder joint may be painful due to excessive capsular stretch. This may be minimized by use of a sling. The sling, however, must hold the humerus elevated *into* the subacromial space and must "seat" the head of the humerus into the glenoid. Figure 49 in Chapter 3 depicts these slings.

If pain is considered to be from the capsular or cuff traction, intraarticular injection of an anesthetic agent with or without steroid can be beneficial. The capsule can be penetrated by injection as indicated in Figure 64. If pain is considered to be related to the coracoid (as verified by local tenderness and pain from the appropriate arm movements) or from the coracohumeral

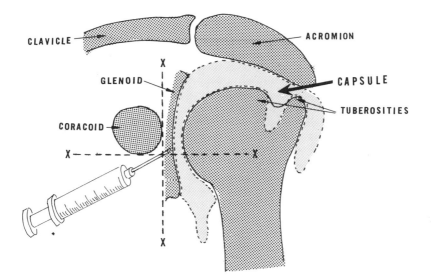

CLAVICLE

ACROMION

GLENOID

CAPSULE

CORACOID

TUBEROSITIES

X

X

X

X

FIGURE 64. Injection technique for intraarticular arthrogram and brisement treatment. The injection site is a point just inferior and lateral to the coracoid process in the vector lines drawn X–X.

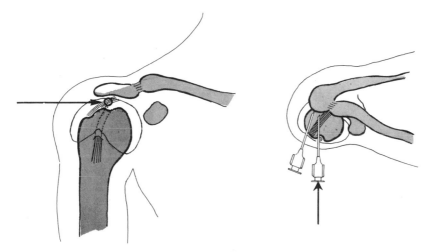

FIGURE 65. Technique for injection treatment of supraspinatus tendinitis. The site of injection is determined by palpating the inferior margin of the acromion: immediately below the greater tuberosity can be located, and the biceps groove immediately medial to the tuberosity can be identified by external-internal rotation of the arm. The tendinitis is injected by entering the superhumeral space and advancing the needle posteriorly, medially, and slightly upward. No obstruction should be encountered.

101

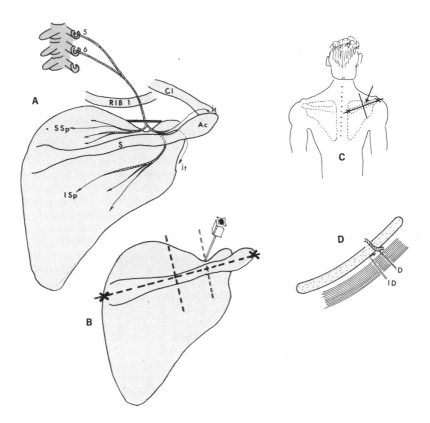

FIGURE 66. Suprascapular nerve block. *A* depicts the origin and course of the nerve. *B,* Clinically, the site of injection is located by measuring between the medial and lateral borders of the spine, dividing the outer one half in thirds, and injecting immediately above the rim of the spine at the inner one third. Staying close to the superior margin of the spine, the needle progresses to touching the spine. After aspiration to make sure no vascular tissues have been encountered, the anesthetic agent is injected. The nerve need not be directly injected as the fluid will reach it via fascial planes.

ligament (tenderness lateral to coracoid, between it and the humerus, and related to restriction of abduction elevation and external rotation), local injection of anesthetic agent and steroid can afford relief. Pain attributed to supraspinatus tendinitis can be reduced by injection of anesthetic agent and steroid or by the use of ultrasound and oral acute inflammatory medications (Fig.

102

65). When pain is recalcitrant, generalized, yet resistant to other modalities used for pain relief, suprascapular nerve block is easily and safely administered (Fig. 66).

The painful shoulder in the spastic hemiplegic has been attributed to spasm and contracture of the subscapularis muscle.[10,11] This muscle is the principal internal rotator of the shoulder and a powerful adductor. When conservative measures fail, surgical release has been found to be effective. Through an anterior deltopectoral approach which preserves the anterior capsule, a block resection of the subscapularis tendon is performed. The pectoralis major tendon is also severed and allowed to reinsert of its own destiny. It is of interest that immediately upon the release of the subscapularis tendon and the pectoralis major tendon *there is no increase in abduction and external rotation* of the arm. The increase is gained by postoperative splinting (Fig. 67) and by active postoperative physical therapy.

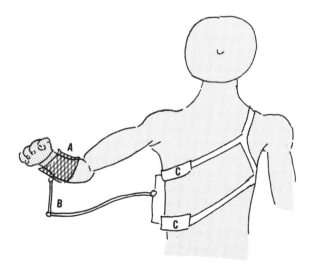

FIGURE 67. Postoperative bracing. After resection of the subscapularis muscle insertion, the arm is held in abducted and external rotation. Forearm band (A) swivels to permit elbow motion. (B) holds arm abducted from body attachment (C). (Modified from Rancho Los Amigos, Calif.)

This includes active self-directed exercises using an overhead pully (Fig. 68) and shoulder exercises (Fig. 69).

In the adhesive capsulitis frozen shoulder, there are many who claim that this condition is self-limited and a *matter of time in spite of treatment*. However, although pain may subside or even disappear, limited range of motion may be an unacceptable residual. Simon[16] has advocated a treatment he terms "infiltration brisement." Under a general anesthetic he inserts the needle into the capsule (as depicted in Fig. 64). With two 50 cc. Luer lock syringes filled with 0.3 percent Xylocaine and 20 mg. triamcino-

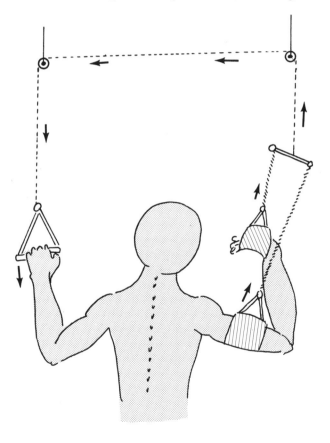

FIGURE 68. Home exercises for painful restricted shoulder. Downward pull by the unaffected arm abducts, elevates, and externally rotates the affected arm.

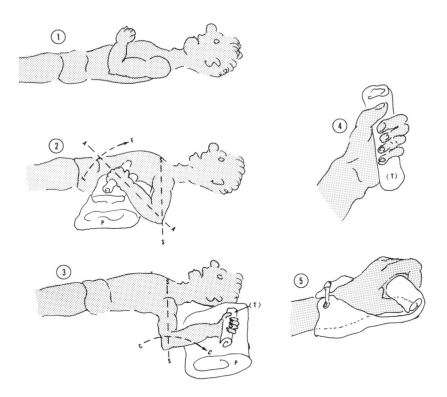

FIGURE 69. Shoulder exercises. With arm abducted to 90° and the hand held with wrist extended (4) and fingers cupped in some extension, the arm is rotated towards overhead position (3). This exercise regains and maintains shoulder range of motion.

lone, he inserts the fluid into the capsule under manual pressure. He uses the maximum pressure that can be exerted upon the syringe manually. At a certain point a "give" is experienced which indicates rupture of the capsule. Active physical therapy, consisting of active and passive range of motion exercises, is initiated, an abduction elevation splint is applied, and the patient is instructed in active exercises. Should there be severe pain following the initial brisement, several more injections into the capsule of the anesthetic-steroid solution are administered.

SUMMARY

The painful shoulder in many ways and with similar causative factors is similar to the nonhemiplegic shoulder. The hemiplegic shoulder that is flail and the one that is spastic present several additional factors that must be considered in diagnosis and treatment. Diagnosis is based on identifying the incriminating tissue and the particular musculoskeletal mechanism, whether it be position or movement, that has initiated the noxious tissue trauma. Treatment is based upon relieving the inflammation or irritation of these tissues and restoring greater range of motion: both active and passive.

REFERENCES

1. Cailliet, R.: Shoulder Pain. F. A. Davis Co., Philadelphia, 1966.
2. Bland, J. H., Merrit, J. A., and Booshey, D. K.: Seminars in arthritis and rheumatism. Arthritis Rheum. 7:21, Aug. 1977.
3. Codman, E. A.: The Shoulder. Todd, Boston, 1934.
4. Hazleman, B. L.: The painful stiff shoulder. Rheumatol. Phys. Med. 2: 413, 1972.
5. Sheldon, P. J. H.: A retrospective study of 102 cases of shoulder pain. Rheumatol. Phys. Med. 2:402, 1972.
6. Boyle, A. C.: Disorders of the shoulder joint. Brit. Med. J. 3:283, 1969.
7. Kerwein, G. A.: Roentgenographic diagnoses of shoulder dysfunction. J.A.M.A. 194:1081, 1965.
8. Steindler, A.: Lecture on the interpretation of pain in orthopedic practice. Charles C Thomas, Springfield, Ill., 1959.
9. Lippmann, R. K.: Frozen shoulder: periarthritis bicipital tenosynovitis. Arch. Surg. 47:283, 1943.
10. Braun, R. M., West, F., Mooney, V., et al.: Surgical treatment of the painful shoulder contracture in the stroke patient. J. Bone Joint Surg. 53A(7):1307, Oct. 1971.
11. Sever, J. W.: Obstetrical paralysis: its etiology, pathology, clinical aspects and treatment with a report of four hundred and seventy cases. A.J. Dis. Child. 12(6):541, Dec. 1916.
12. Caldwell, C. B., Wilson, D. J., and Braun, R. M.: Evaluation and treatment of the upper extremity in the hemiplegic stroke patient. Clin. Orthop. 63:69, March–April 1969.
13. Neviaser, J. S.: Adhesive capsulitis of the shoulder: a study of the pathological findings in periarthritis of the shoulder. J. Bone Joint Surg. 27:211, 1945.
14. Moskowitz, E., and Porter, J. T.: Peripheral nerve lesions in upper extremity in hemiplegic patients. N. Engl. J. Med. 269:776, 1963.
15. Travell, J., and Rinzler, S.: The myofascial genesis of pain. Postgrad. Med. 2:425, 1952.
16. Simon, W. H.: Soft tissue disorders of the shoulder. Orthopedic Clin. No. Am. 6(2):521, April 1975.

CHAPTER 6

Shoulder-Hand-Finger Syndrome

Circulation of the upper extremity is:

1. Arterial. By cardiac pumping action and vascular tone plus gravity, the circulation goes to the distal portion of the extremities.
2. Venous and lymphatic. Pumping action of the muscles of the hand and arm forces fluid in a centripetal direction through numerous valves in the venous system. The pumping action constitutes pressure exerted intermittently upon the veins and lympathics by the tension of the muscles, the fascia, the skin, aided by gravity from repeated elevation of the arm above cardiac level.

The major pumps are located in the axilla and the hand. These pumps require repeated movement through an adequate range of motion of the shoulder girdle (principally the glenohumeral joint) and frequent clenching and release of the wrist and fingers. Elevation of the entire arm above cardiac level facilitates centripetal circulation by the addition of gravity (Fig. 70). Most of the arterial supply is located in the volar (flexor or palmar) aspect of the hand, whereas most of the venous lymphatic drainage is in the *dorsal* aspect. Failure or impairment of the pumps in the shoulder or the hand for any reason leads to a painful disabling condition that has become known as the *shoulder-hand-finger syndrome*. Either of the pumps, the shoulder or the

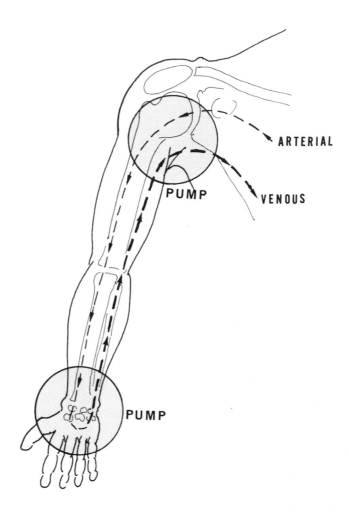

ARTERIAL

PUMP

VENOUS

PUMP

FIGURE 70.   Venous lymphatic pumps of the upper extremity.

hand, may initiate the syndrome and remain a single or a double involvement. The onset of one ultimately involves the other.

The shoulder component of the syndrome involves limitation of range of motion in which the pump becomes deficient and the arm becomes dependent. Immobilization of the shoulder may be caused by hemiplegia, both the flail and spastic phases, due to pain from peritendinitis, capsulitis, or biceps tendinitis, or from fracture, dislocation, hemarthrosis, and so forth. Pain may be referred from cervical radiculitis or cardiac anginal pain. Any painful or limiting affliction of the arm can be implicated. Prolonged holding of the arm in a sling at the side for any reason may initiate the syndrome. Immobilization of the arm from stroke has been discussed in Chapter 4. There is restricted abduction, elevation, and rotation of the arm at the glenohumeral joint with secondary changes in the soft tissues about and within the joint. The hand and fingers become immobile due to flaccidity, spasticity, loss of sensation, or mere dependency.

The hand-finger component, whether primary or secondary, first manifests itself as edema. This edema is predominantly noted on the dorsum of the hand and usually over the metacarpophalangeal and proximal interphalangeal joints (Fig. 71). The skin over the knuckles becomes puffy and loses its normal creased appearance. The hand at first becomes painful and boggy. The

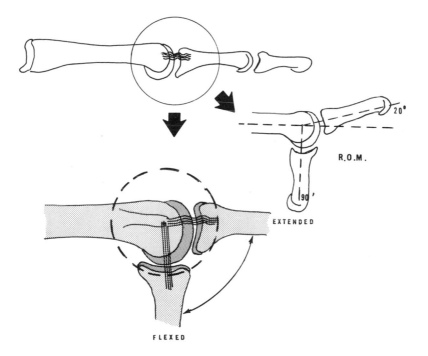

FIGURE 71. Normal flexion-extension of metacarpophalangeal joints. Due to the elliptical shape of the head of the metacarpals, the collateral ligaments are slack with finger extension and taut when the fingers are flexed.

109

extensor tendons become elevated by the edema which gradually prevents flexion of the joints. The collateral ligaments that must elongate to permit flexion of the metacarpophalangeal joint become shortened and thus prevent or limit full flexion (Fig. 72). If the wrist is fixed in flexion, the fingers become extended through tenodesis action and further flexion is prevented. Less pumping action is possible consequently. The skin gradually be-

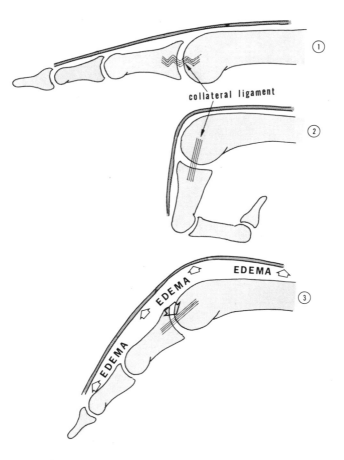

FIGURE 72. Finger changes in hand-shoulder syndrome. *1*, Normal extension of metacarpophalangeal joint with relaxed collateral ligament. *2*, Normal flexion of metacarpophalangeal joint with the collaterals becoming taut. *3*, Edema on dorsum of hand elevates the extensor tendons and prevents flexion. The collateral ligaments are never fully elongated and develop contracture. This further limits the "pump action" of the flexion of the hand.

110

comes shiny and atrophic. The edema, containing protein, converts into a diffuse cobweb-like scar tissue that adheres to the tendons and joint capsules and prevents further movement. The joints undergo disuse atrophy of the cartilage with thickening of the capsule. Disuse osteoporosis of the bones gradually develops. The usual hand posture in the shoulder-hand-finger syndrome is stiffening of the metacarpophalangeal joint in extension which, by tenodesis action of the flexors, flexes the interphalangeal joints. This hand resembles the *intrinsic minus hand*. Occasionally, the interphalangeal joints become fixed in extension and the metacarpophalangeal joint remains flexed thus resembling an *intrinsic plus hand* (Fig. 73).

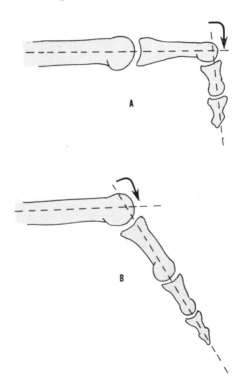

FIGURE 73. Hand patterns. *A*, Depicts the hand that resembles the "intrinsic minus hand." The proximal phalanx remains extended with tenodesis action flexing the distal phalanges. *B*, This hand resembles the "intrinsic minus hand," with all phalanges extended but with the metacarpophalangeal joint flexed.

The evolution of the shoulder-hand-finger syndrome can be itemized in the following sequence (Fig. 74):

1. Impairment of the hand-arm-shoulder venous and lymphatic circulation.
2. Shoulder limitation from numerous causes leading to ultimate contracture (frozen shoulder).

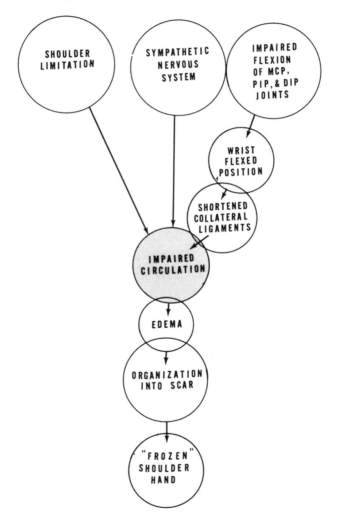

FIGURE 74. Sequences leading to frozen shoulder-hand-finger syndrome.

3. Metacarpophalangeal limitation due to edema and restricting, contracted collateral ligaments.
4. Wrist in a restricted, flexed position.
5. Sympathetic nervous system involvement.

Sympathetic nervous system involvement may be totally absent, initially absent, or may be primary in the causation of the shoulder-hand-finger syndrome. Some deny the necessity of this component (Moberg[1]) based on the fact that the syndrome is rarely seen in people who are less than 40 years old, which is when sympathetic nervous system abnormalities are most prevalent. Causes considered necessary for sympathetic nervous system involvement are frequently not present. When present, the resultant clinical entity is termed *reflex sympathetic dystrophy syndrome* or *causalgia*.

Reflex sympathetic dystrophy syndrome has the following classic signs and symptoms:

1. Pain and swelling in an extremity
2. Trophic skin changes of that extremity which include:
   a. Skin atrophy
   b. Skin pigmentary changes
   c. Hyperhidrosis
   d. Hypertrichosis
   e. Nail changes
3. Signs and symptoms of vasomotor instability
4. Pain and limited range of motion of the ipsilateral shoulder
5. Precipitating events such as stroke, trauma, myocardial infarct, and so on.

Most reflex sympathetic dystrophy syndromes are unilateral but 25 percent (20 to 35 percent) are bilateral. Studies of reflex dystrophy by oscillography, plethysmography, skin temperature, and venous gas determinations reveal increased blood flow and increased venous oxygen. In reflex sympathetic dystrophy syndrome, there are *no* characteristic pathologic tissue changes. Ul-

113

timately, there is radiologic evidence of periarticular soft tissue swelling and patchy osteoporosis, but these changes are similar to changes noted in prolonged immobilization.[2]

The shoulder-hand-finger syndrome, which is a variant of the reflex sympathetic dystrophy syndrome, has been considered to evolve into three stages. These stages need not be in the same sequence, but the third stage is usually the residual stage. The stages are also not necessarily so specific or as clearly delineated as stated.

Stage I. Limited shoulder range of motion with or without pain. The hand has swelling limited initially to the dorsum of the fingers, knuckles, and wrist. Edema is not usually of the pitting variety but is firm. The skin loses its normal wrinkles and becomes shiny. Full flexion of the fingers and all their joints becomes limited. The wrist tends to assume a flexed posture. The skin of the hand may be pale and cool or assume a pink hue. The skin is usually moist with small bubbles of perspiration. In certain cases, the skin is excessively hypersensitive to touch, pressure, movement, or temperature variations. The elbow usually shows no limitation or pain. The wrist is usually exquisitely painful when extended and also has dorsal edema and tenderness.

Stage II. Shoulder pain subsides and shoulder range may increase. Residual restriction of movement in both the active and passive ranges may persist, but this limitation is usually less painful. Edema of the hand subsides but the fingers become stiffer. The skin assumes a pale atrophic appearance. Hair appears courser, as do the nails. Sensitivity decreases. Osteoporosis can now be visualized on x-ray.

Stage III. There is progressive atrophy of the bones, skin, and muscles. Limitation of hands, wrists, and fingers increases leaving the hand painless but in a useless, atrophied, clawed position.

In the hemiplegic patient, the shoulder-hand-finger syndrome may occur with either a flail shoulder or a spastic shoulder so that limited range of motion is not a prerequisite. The fact that the shoulder is flail and the arm cannot be actively elevated, forward flexed, or abducted to place the hand in a functional

114

antigravity position is of undoubted significance. A painful flail shoulder may develop into a shoulder-hand-finger syndrome.

The time between stroke and the first symptoms of shoulder-hand-finger syndrome has been estimated in the following graph:[4,5]

Months	Percentage of Patients
0–1	0
1–2	28
2–3	37
3–4	16
4–5	17
5–6	2

THEORIES OF ETIOLOGY OF PAIN

Initial causalgic pain is mediated through the large delta fibers which transmit brief, sharp, pricking, localized pain which, when elicited, promptly causes withdrawal. The secondary pain is delayed and mediated through the small diameter fibers that are slow conducting. This is the pain that is persistent and of a burning quality. In causalgia, the macroscopic and microscopic appearance of the involved nerve lesions is not different from lesions which do not cause burning pain.

Electrical stimulation of the distal end of the divided nerves in a peripheral nerve injury with causalgia releases neurokinin, a substance that is a vasodilator. Neurokinin, which can be retrieved from the tissues will cause a burning pain when injected into normal tissues. In causalgia, it is probable that neurokinin is liberated, but this has not been verified.

TREATMENT

Interruption of the sympathetic fibers stops the burning pain. Benefit, however, may be temporary. More permanent benefit from sympathetic intervention can be prognosticated as:

1. Good
   a. If one block gives total relief
   b. If one block reduces pain to a tolerable level
   c. If the first block is effective with each subsequent block being "better"
2. Poor
   a. If the first block is effective but each subsequent block is less effective
   b. If the block is only effective during the duration of the anesthetic agent but no residual benefit remains when the anesthetic agent wears off

Administration of a stellate chemical block requires a thorough anatomic knowledge and the ability and equipment to administer resuscitation and to deal with the possibility of an adverse reaction. It is claimed that 20 percent of patients receiving a stellate block experience an adverse reaction. Many patients also may refuse repeated supraclavicular injections (Fig. 75).

If the decision is made not to administer a stellate chemical block, oral or intramuscular steroids can be beneficially administered. The usual dosage is triamcinolone, 100 mg. daily (cortisone 200 mg. daily) for 14 to 16 days. The precautions are determining the presence of diabetes and/or hypertension. Ingestions of antacids are usually given in divided doses to avoid gastric irritation.

As there is considered to be a personality factor in the development of sympathetic reflex dystrophy,[5] this must be taken into consideration by use of reassurance, explanation, operant conditioning, and psychotropic drugs. These personality factors are stated to be in the patient who:

1. Is passively apathetic.
2. Demonstrates muscular tension and ability.
3. Is hyperemotional with hyperactive vasomotor responses.
4. Has a dependent personality.
5. Is intolerant to pain.[5]

116

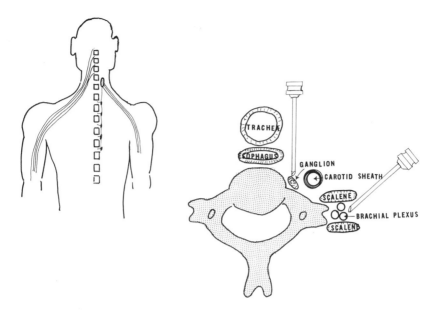

FIGURE 75. Technique of stellate ganglion or brachial plexus block. For a stellate ganglion nerve block, the trachea is moved to one side and the needle enters between it and the carotid artery to the vertebral body. The needle then is moved slightly lateral to the body and 3 to 5 cc. of the anesthetic agent is administered. Aspiration must always precede infiltration of the anesthetic agent.

In addition to the chemical sympathetic blocks and oral steroids or intramuscular steroids, all the physical factors that have been eluded to in the previous chapters such as maintaining range of motion and keeping the arm elevated, must be employed. As much as possible, active and passive range of motion at the shoulder and active and passive range of motion of the fingers at all the joints (the metacarpophalangeal joints and proximal and distal interphalangeal joints) must be maintained by repeated flexion and extension. This necessitates attempting full or close to full range of motion.

Vasoconstrictive techniques such as compression dressings like Ace bandages, wrapping the fingers with twine from the distal portion of the finger to the proximal, or use of a Jobst vasopneumatic compressive instrument are usually of value (Fig. 76). The need for continued, daily, active and passive range

117

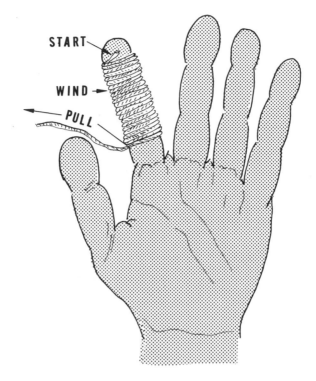

FIGURE 76. Removal of finger edema. Each finger is firmly wrapped with a heavy twine, beginning at the tip and moving towards the webbing. This procedure should be performed several times daily and can frequently be done by the patient using his uninvolved upper extremity.

of motion and elevation of the arm above heart level is mandatory, as is the need for a constant pressure dressing. The sleeve of Johnstone as depicted in Figure 41 is usually not of significant compression to facilitate venous and lymphatic return. An Ace bandage, properly applied beginning from distal to proximal, is of great value as is a hand or machine pumped vasopneumatic sleeve. In a hospital setting or in a well controlled home setting, elevation of the arm with a Webril dressing of the hand slung from an overhead bed support which keeps the arm in an elevated position with the shoulder forward flexed and abducted is of great value for preventing edema. It should be used for numerous hours of the day and at night during the sleeping hours

118

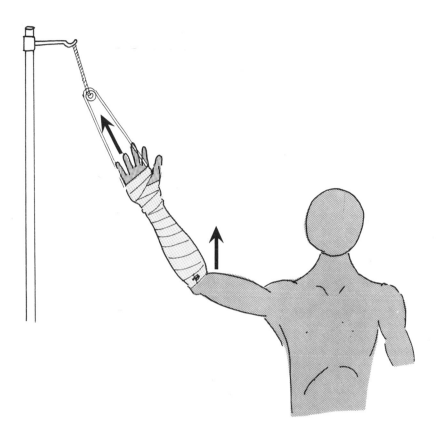

FIGURE 77. Antigravity treatment of the edematous extremity. The hand and arm are wrapped with an elastic bandage, from distal to proximal. The hand held by the webrill is then suspended overhead. This position drains the edema and maintains shoulder range of motion with the elbow extended.

(Fig. 77). As soon as any active motion is possible or the patient is capable of using the uninvolved arm to elevate, massage, and range the joints of the hand, this should be instituted.

REFERENCES

1. Moberg, E.: The shoulder-hand-finger syndrome as a whole. Surg. Clin. N. Am. 40(2):367, April 1960.
2. Kozin, F., McCarty, D. J., Sims, S., et al.: The reflex sympathetic dystrophy syndrome. Am. J. Med. 60:321, March 1976.

119

3. Davis, S. W., Petrillo, C. R., Eichberg, R. D., et al.: Shoulder-hand syndrome in a hemiplegic population—a five-year retrospective study. Arch. Phys. Med. Rehabil. 58:353, Aug. 1977.
4. Lusskin, R., Grynbaum, B. B., and Dhie, R. S.: Rehabilitation surgery on adult spastic hemiplegia. Clin. Orthop. 63:32, 1969.
5. Coventry, M. B.: Problem of painful shoulder. J.A.M.A. 151(3):177, Jan. 1953.

CHAPTER 7

Brachial Plexus Injury

Concomitant musculoskeletal and neuromuscular complications can obscure the hemiplegia. A brachial plexus traction injury during the flail phase, from an inadvertent injury caused by a spouse, a nurse, or a therapist, or from faulty position of the patient may be present and not be recognized. The injury may have occurred during the early phase of impaired consciousness. This should be suspected when the normal pattern of recovery is altered. Normally, the proximal position of the extremity recovers more rapidly than does the intrinsic function of the hand. This sequence can be reversed in a brachial plexus injury. Abnormal EMG changes, which test lower motor neuron function, should indicate peripheral nerve or brachial plexus injury and not be evident in hemiplegia.

Atrophy, or masked paresis of the upper muscles of the arm (shoulder girdle, deltoid, triceps) with fair to good recovery of hand-fingers, indicates the possibility of a peripheral nerve injury. Finding fibrillation or polyphasic units implicates a specific peripheral nerve or injury to the brachial plexus. Specific myotome changes are inconsistent with the hemiplegic patient.

Flaccidity is difficult to differentiate from the flail aspect of hemiplegia with lower motor neuron involvement. Atrophy is usually not marked in the stroke patient. Failure to follow the normal recovery pattern, i.e., initial recovery of the shoulder,

121

followed by the elbow and wrist, lastly, finger extensors and thumb opposition, indicates the strong possibility of brachial plexus traction injury. Deviation from the usual hemiplegic arm pattern in which the patient usually has an adducted, internally rotated shoulder, flexion of the elbow and wrist, and fingers flexed over an adducted thumb should raise suspicion of a complication neuropathy.

In a random sampling of extremities of hemiplegic patients, fibrillations have been found in 56.8 percent and positive sharp waves in 69.6 percent. This has varied with the time after onset of stroke that the EMG was performed. The greatest number of abnormalities was noted 4 1/2 weeks after onset of hemiplegia. Fibrillation was found twice as frequently in the upper extremities as in the lower, but no segmental or peripheral nerve patterns could be discerned. There were no nerve conductor abnormalities in the patients with nerve damage. The basis for these findings could not be determined insofar as the anterior horn cell has never been considered involved in hemiplegia. Anterior horn cell changes have been reported in spinal cord injuries, however, attributed to the combined absence of descending motor impulses and sensory impulses upon the anterior horn cell.

The importance of discovering the presence of a peripheral nerve injury or a brachial plexus traction injury is that:

1. Treatment should be directed to the peripheral nerve injury.
2. Treatment techniques may differ for the peripheral nerve damage and not be applicable to the hemiplegic therapy.
3. Prognosis and rate of recovery vary tremendously.

Bibliography

Amato, A., Hermsmeyer, C., and Kleinman, K.: Use of electro-myographic feedback to increase inhibitory control of spastic muscles. Phys. Ther. 53(10):1063, Oct. 1973.

Amick, L. D., Gilmer, W. J., and Sutton, F. D.: The holistic approach to the shoulder-hand syndrome. South. Med. J. 59:161, Feb. 1969.

Anderson, T. P., and Kottke, F. J.: Stroke rehabilitation: a reconsideration of some common attitudes. Arch. Phys. Med. Rehabil. 59(4):175, April 1978.

Antonio, C. T., Tso, M. L., and Roper, R. B.: Vest sling for reducing pain. Am. J. Occup. Ther. 31(3):174, 1977.

Bobath, K., and Bobath, B.: Spastic paralysis. Treatment by use of reflex inhibition. Brit. J. Phys. Med. 13(6):121, June 1950.

Cailliet, R.: Shoulder Pain. F. A. Davis Co., Philadelphia, 1966.

Cailliet, R.: Soft Tissue Pain and Disability. F. A. Davis Co., Philadelphia, 1977.

Chokroverty, S., and Medina, J.: Electrophysiological study of hemiplegia. Arch. Neurol. 35:360, June 1978.

Cobb, C. R., deVries, H. A., Urban, R. T., et al.: Electrical activity in muscle pain. Am. J. Phys. Med. 54(2):80, 1975.

Codman, E. A.: The Shoulder. Thomas Todd Co., Boston, 1934.

Coventry, M. B.: Problem of painful shoulder. JAMA 151(3): 177, Jan. 1953.

Davis, S. W., Petrillo, C. R., Eichberg, R. D., et al.: Shoulder-hand syndrome in a hemiplegic population: a five year retrospective study. Arch. Phys. Med. Rehabil. 58:353, Aug. 1977.

DeVore, G. L., and Denny, E.: A sling to prevent a subluxed shoulder. Am. J. Occup. Ther. 24(8):580, 1970.

DiPalma, A. F.: Surgery of the Shoulder. J. B. Lippincott Co., Philadelphia, 1950.

Dontigney, R. L.: Passive shoulder exercises. Phys. Ther. 50 (12):1707, Dec. 1970.

deTakats, G.: Sympathetic reflex dystrophy. Med. Clin. No. Am. 49:117, 1965.

Fields, W. S., and Moossy, J.: Stroke: Diagnosis and Management. Warren H. Green Inc., St. Louis, 1973.

Fields, W. S., and Spencer, W. A.: Stroke Rehabilitation: Basic Concepts and Research Trends. Warren H. Green, Inc., St. Louis, 1967.

Fitzgerald-Finch, O. P., and Gibson, I. I.: Subluxation of the shoulder in hemiplegia. Age Ageing 4(1):16, Feb. 1975.

Glick, E. N.: Reflex dystrophy (algoneurodystrophy): results of treatment by corticosteroids. Rheumatol. Rehabil. 12:84, 1973.

Goldkamp, O.: Electromyography and nerve conduction. Studies in 116 patients with hemiplegia. 48:59, Feb. 1967.

Hausmanowa-Petrusewicz, I.: Interaction is simultaneous motor functions. AMA Arch. Neurol. Psychiat. 81:173, 1959.

Hollinshead, W. H.: Functional Anatomy of the Limbs, ed. 5. W. B. Saunders Co., Philadelphia, 1952.

Inaba, M. K., and Piorkowski, M.: Ultrasound in treatment of painful shoulder in patients with hemiplegia. Phys. Ther. 52(7):737, July 1972.

Inman, V. T., Saunders, J. B., and Abbott, L. C.: Observations of the function of the shoulder joint. J. Bone Joint Surg. 26:11, Jan. 1944.

124

Johnson, H. E., and Garton, W. H.: Muscle reeducation in hemiplegia by use of electromyographic devices. Arch. Phys. Med. Rehabil. 54:320, July 1973.

Juilliard, C.: La coracoidite. Helv. Med. Acta 1:88, 1934.

Juilliard, C.: La coracoidite. Rev. Med. Suisse Romande 53 (12):737, Oct. 1933.

Kaplan, P. E., Meredith, J., Taft, G., et al.: Stroke and brachial plexus injury: a difficult problem. Arch. Phys. Med. Rehabil. 58:415, Sept. 1977.

Knott, M., and Voss, D.: Proprioceptive Neuromuscular Facilitation: Patterns and Techniques, ed. 2. Harper & Row, New York, 1968.

Kopell, H. R., and Thompson, W. A. L.: Pain and the frozen shoulder. Surg. Gynecol. Obstet. 109:92, 1959.

Leffert, R. D.: Brachial-plexus injuries: medical progress. New Engl. J. Med. 291(20):1059, Nov. 1974.

Lehmann, J. F., Warren, C. G., and Scham, S. M.: Therapeutic heat and cold. Clin. Orthop. 99:207, March–April, 1974.

Licht, S. (ed): Stroke and Its Rehabilitation. Eliz. Licht Pub., New Haven, 1975.

Lusskin, R., Nemonaitis, J., Umer, J., et al.: Corrective surgery in adult hemiplegia. Arch. Phys. Med. Rehabil. 49:437, Aug. 1968.

Meyer, G. A., and Fields, H. L.: Causalgia treated by selective large nerve fibre stimulation of peripheral nerve. Brain 95:163, 1972.

Moseley, H. F.: Disorders of the shoulder. Clin. Symp. 11:3, May–July 1959.

Moseley, H. F.: Shoulder Lesions. Churchill Livingstone, New York, 1969.

Moseley, H. F., and Goldie, I.: The arterial pattern of the rotator cuff. J. Bone Joint Surg. 45–B:4, Nov. 1963.

Moskowitz, E.: Complications in rehabilitation of hemiplegic patients. Med. Clin. No. Amer. 53(3):547, May, 1969.

Moskowitz, E., and Porter, J. J.: Peripheral nerve lesions in the upper extremity in hemiplegic patients. New Engl. J. Med. 269:776, Oct. 1963.

Mossman, P. L.: A Problem Oriented Approach to Stroke Rehabilitation. Charles C Thomas, Publisher, Springfield, Ill., 1976.

Mroczek, N., Halpern, D., and McHugh, R.: Electromyographic retraining in hemiplegia. Arch. Phys. Med. Rehabil. 59 (6):258, June 1978.

Nepomuceno, C. S.: Shoulder arthrography in hemiplegic shoulder. Arch. Phys. Med. Rehabil. 55:49, Feb. 1974.

Omer, G., and Thomas, S.: Treatment of causalgia: review of cases at Brook General Hospital. Tex. Med. 67:93, Jan. 1971.

Pender, J. W.: Basic concepts about shoulder-arm syndrome. JAMA 169(8):795, Feb. 1959.

Richards, R. L.: Causalgia: a centennial review. Arch. Neurol. 16:339, April 1967.

Steindler, A.: Kinesiology of the Human Body. Charles C Thomas, Publisher, Springfield, Ill., 1955.

Stern, P., McDowell, F., Miller, J., et al.: Effects of facilitation exercise techniques in strike rehabilitation. Arch. Phys. Med. Rehab. 51:526, 1970.

Sternschein, M. J., Myers, S. J., Frewin, D. B., et al.: Causalgia. Arch. Phys. Med. Rehabil. 56:58, Feb. 1975.

Steverson, B.: The Steverson sling for the flaccid hemiplegic. Am. J. Occup. Ther. 27(1):44, 1973.

Stockmeyer, S. A.: An interpretation of the approach of Rood to the treatment of neuromuscular dysfunction. Am. J. Phys. Med. 46(1):900, 1967.

Taketomi, Y.: Observations on subluxation of the shoulder joint in hemiplegia. Phys. Ther. 55(1):39, Jan. 1975.

Tavernick, L., et al.: La section des nerfs articularies dans le traitment des arthritis sechs douloureuses de l'epaule. Lyon Chir. 38:6, Nov.–Dec. 1943.

126

Index

ABDUCTION, shoulder, 34–35, 42–43, 48
Acromioclavicular joint, 44–46
Acromioclavicular lesion, 95
Acromiocoracoid arch, 12–13
Adhesive capsulitis, 104–105
Agnosia in spastic stage, 76
Anastomosis, critical zone of, 27–28
Anatomy, functional
    acromioclavicular joint, 44–46
    acromiocoracoid arch, 12–13
    biceps brachii, 49–50
    biceps tendon, 16–17
    bursae, 26
    circumflex (axillary) nerve, 27
    coracoacromial arch, 19
    coracoclavicular ligament, 44–46
    coracohumeral ligament, 20
    costoclavicular ligament, 46–47
    deltoid muscle, 32–34
    foramen of Weitbrecht, 18
    glenohumeral joint, 11–18
    glenohumeral ligaments, 18
    glenoid fossa, 13
    glenoid labrum, 13
    infraspinatus muscle, 23–25, 34
    latissimus dorsi, 41
    levator scapula, 39
    musculotendinous cuff, 20–22
    pectoralis major, 40–41
    pectoralis minor, 41–42
    rhomboid major, 39
    rhomboid minor, 39
    rotator cuff, 20–22
    scapula, 12, 36–42
    serratus anterior, 39
    shoulder, 11–53
    sternoclavicular joint, 46–47
    subscapularis muscle, 26
    suprahumeral joint, 11–12, 18–20
    suprascapular nerve, 27
    supraspinatus muscle, 22–23, 34
    suspensory ligaments, 20
    teres minor, 25–26, 34
    trapezius muscle, 37–39
Antagonist, relaxation of, 79
Associated reactions in spastic stage, 76
Astereognosis in spastic stage, 76

BICEPS brachii, 49–50
Biceps muscle
    lesions of, 96
    mechanism of, 49–52
Biceps tendon, 16–17
Bicipital tendinitis syndrome, 94
    painful shoulder and, 95–96
Bicipital tenosynovitis, 96
Bilateral training, 83
Biofeedback in muscle reeducation, 79, 84–85
Bobath's muscular weakness concepts, 78
Body rolling, 60–61
Brachial plexus injury, 121–122
Brachial plexus traction, 98–99
Bursae, 26

CALCIUM deposits in painful shoulder, 90–91
Capsule, glenohumeral, 16–18
Causalgia, 113, 115
Central nervous system, 3
Circulation, upper extremity, 107
Circumflex (axillary) nerve, 27
Codman scapulohumeral rhythm, 35

Coracoacromial arch, 19
Coracoclavicular ligament, 44–46
Coracohumeral ligament, 20
Coracoiditis, 96–97
Costoclavicular ligament, 46–47
Critical zone of vascular anastomosis, 27–28

DELTOID muscle
  anatomy of, 32–34
  flail extremity and, 62–63
Drugs for painful shoulder, 99–100

ELECTROMYOGRAPHIC feedback in muscle reeducation and, 84–85
Elevation, shoulder, 48–49
Exercises
  painful shoulder and, 100
  sitting balance, 79
Extremity
  flail. *See* Flail extremity.
  upper. *See* Upper extremity.

FLACCID stage, 55–71
Flail extremity, 55–63
  body rolling and, 60–61
  deltoid in, 62–63
  glenohumeral joint in, 60
  initiating reflex activity of, 55–56
  labyrinthine reflexes and, 56–58
  positions to avoid with, 58–59
  proper positioning of, 58–60
  sensory feedback and, 56
  sitting up and weight bearing with, 61–62
  tonic neck reflexes and, 56
  treatment of, 58–63
Foramen of Weitbrecht, 18
Frozen shoulder, 20
  causes of, 97
  infiltration brisement in, 104–105

GLENOHUMERAL joint
  capsule of, 16–18
  functional anatomy of, 11–18
  incongruous, 14–15
  manual mobilization of, 60
  movement of, 30–36

musculature of, 20–26
stability of, 30–31, 64
Glenohumeral ligaments, 18
Glenoid fossa, 13
Glenoid labrum, 13

HAND
  intrinsic minus, 111
  intrinsic plus, 111
Hemiparesis, scapulohumeral rhythm and, 43
Hemiplegia, 1–10
  neuropathology in, 2–4
  typical arm pattern in, 75
  upper extremity function in, 4–8

INFILTRATION brisement in adhesive capsulitis, 104–105
Infraspinatus muscle, 23–25, 34
Intraarticular injection for painful shoulder, 100–103
Intrinsic minus hand, 111
Intrinsic plus hand, 111

JOINT(S). *See also individual joints.*
  congruous, 15
  incongruous, 14–15

LABYRINTHINE reflexes in flail extremity, 56–58
Latissimus dorsi, 41
Levator scapula, 39
Ligaments. *See individual ligaments.*

MENTAL status investigation in muscle reeducation, 85
Modalities in painful shoulder, 100
Muscular weakness, Bobaths' concepts of, 78
Muscle reeducation. *See* Reeducation, muscular.
Musculotendinous cuff, 20–22

NERVE(S). *See individual nerves.*
Nerve supply of shoulder, 27–29
Neuropathology in hemiplegia, 2–4

PAINFUL shoulder, 89–106
  acromioclavicular lesion in, 95
  bicipital tendinitis and, 95–96

128

PAINFUL shoulder—*Continued*
brachial plexus traction and, 98–99
calcium deposits in, 90–91
coracoiditis and, 96–97
diagnosis in, 99
examination of, 91–92
radiologic examination of, 92–95
tendonitis in, 90
treatment of, 99–105
  drugs in, 99–100
  exercises in, 100
  intraarticular injection in, 100–103
  modalities in, 100
  sling in, 100
  subscapularis release in, 103–104
Pectoralis major, 40–41
Pectoralis minor, 41–42
Personality factor in shoulder-hand-finger syndrome, 116
Position of patient during treatment, 56–58
Positioning of flail extremity, 58–60
Posture control, 8
Prognostic factors, negative, 85–86

RADIOLOGIC examination of painful shoulder, 92–95
Range of motion, full recovery of, 7
Recovery
  full range of motion and, 7
  sequence of, 4–5
  spontaneous, 4–5
    percentages in, 7
  stages of, 6–7
Reeducation, muscular
  biofeedback and, 79, 84–85
  electromyographic feedback and, 84–85
  mental status investigation and, 85
  relaxation and, 80–84
  spastic stage and, 79–86
Reflexes
  labyrinthine, flail extremity and, 56–58

tonic neck
  flail extremity and, 56
  spastic stage and, 73–74
  supraspinal, 8
Reflex activity in flail extremity, 55–56
Reflex sympathetic dystrophy syndrome, 113
Relaxation
  of antagonist, 79
  muscle reeducation and, 80–84
Rhomboid major, 39
Rhomboid minor, 39
Rood sling, 68
Rotator cuff, 20–22

SCAPULA
  anatomy of, 12
  movement of, 36–42
Scapulohumeral joint, 12. *See also* Glenohumeral joint.
  movement of, 42–43
Scapulohumeral rhythm, 31
  hemiparesis and, 43
Sensory feedback in flail extremity, 56
Sensory impairment in spastic stage, 76
Serratus anterior, 39
Shoulder
  abduction of, 34–35, 42–43, 48
  forward flexion of, 35–36
  frozen. *See* Frozen shoulder.
  functional anatomy of, 11–53
  nerve supply to, 27–29
  painful, 89–106. *See also* Painful shoulder.
  subluxation of, 63–68. *See also* Subluxation of shoulder.
Shoulder blade, 12. *See also* Scapula.
Shoulder girdle
  abduction of, 48
  composite movements of, 47–49
  overhead elevation of, 48–49
Shoulder-hand-finger syndrome, 107–120
  edema of hand in, 109–111
  evolution of, 112–113
  hand-finger component of, 109–111

Shoulder-hand-finger syndrome— *Continued*
pain etiology in, 115
shoulder component of, 108–109
stages in, 114
sympathetic nervous system and, 113
time between stroke and, 115
treatment of, 115–119
personality factor in, 116
stellate chemical block in, 116
vasoconstrictive techniques in, 117–118
Sitting balance exercises in spastic stage, 79
Sitting up with flail extremity, 61–62
Sling
painful shoulder and, 100
subluxation of shoulder and, 67–68
Spastic stage, 73–87
agnosia and, 76
associated reactions in, 76
astereognosis in, 76
extensor synergy in, 74–75
flexor synergies in, 74–75
muscles initially affected in, 79
muscle reeducation in, 79–86
sensory impairment in, 76
sitting balance exercises and, 79
tonic neck reflexes in, 73–74
trunk movements in, 75
Spasticity, Bobath's muscular weakness concepts and, 78
Stability, glenohumeral, 30–31, 64
Stellate chemical block in shoulder-hand-finger syndrome, 116
Sternoclavicular joint
anatomy of, 46–47
motion of, 49
Stroke syndrome, 1
Subluxation of shoulder, 63–68
causation of, 65
diagnosis of, 65
sling in, 67–68
treatment of, 67–68
Subscapularis muscle
anatomy of, 26
release of, 103–104

Suprahumeral joint, 11–12, 18–20
Suprascapular nerve, 27
Supraspinal tonic neck reflexes, 8
Supraspinatus muscle, 22–23, 34
Suspensory ligaments, 20
Sympathetic nervous system
in shoulder-hand-finger syndrome, 113
Synergy
development of, 7–8
extensor, 74–75
flexor, 74–75

TENDON(S). *See individual tendons.*
Tendonitis, 90
Teres minor, 25–26, 34
Thoracoscapulohumeral articulation, 11
Tonic neck reflexes
flail extremity and, 56
spastic stage and, 73–74
supraspinal, 8
Training, bilateral, 83
Trapezius muscle, 37–39
Treatment
of flail extremity, 58–63
position of patient during, 56–58
pros and cons of, 2
Trunk movements in spastic stage, 75
Two point discrimination, 7

UPPER extremity
circulation of, 107
extensor synergies of, 74–75
flexor synergies of, 74–75
function of, 4–8
influencing factors in, 4
sequence of recovery of, 4–5
stages of recovery of, 6–7
synergistic patterns in, 7–8

VASOCONSTRICTIVE techniques in shoulder-hand-finger syndrome, 117–118

WEAKNESS, muscular, Bobath's concepts of, 78
Weight bearing, flail extremity and, 61–62